T0348629

Education and Professional Development in Rheumatology

Editors

KARINA D. TORRALBA
JAMES D. KATZ

RHEUMATIC DISEASE CLINICS OF NORTH AMERICA

www.rheumatic.theclinics.com

Consulting Editor
MICHAEL H. WEISMAN

February 2020 • Volume 46 • Number 1

ELSEVIER

1600 John F. Kennedy Boulevard ● Suite 1800 ● Philadelphia, Pennsylvania, 19103-2899
http://www.theclinics.com

RHEUMATIC DISEASE CLINICS OF NORTH AMERICA Volume 46, Number 1
February 2020 ISSN 0889-857X, ISBN 13: 978-0-323-69569-5

Editor: Lauren Boyle
Developmental Editor: Casey Potter

Rheumatic Disease Clinics of North America (ISSN 0889-857X) is published quarterly by Elsevier Inc., 360 Park Avenue South, New York, NY 10010-1710. Months of issue are February, May, August, and November. Business and editorial offices: 1600 John F. Kennedy Boulevard, Suite 1800, Philadelphia, PA 19103-2899. Periodicals postage paid at New York, NY and additional mailing offices. Subscription prices are USD 362.00 per year for US individuals, USD 777.00 per year for US institutions, USD 100.00 per year for US students and residents, USD 427.00 per year for Canadian individuals, USD 971.00 per year for Canadian institutions, USD 100.00 per year for Canadian students/residents, USD 465.00 per year for international individuals, USD 971.00 per year for international institutions, and USD 230.00 per year for foreign students/residents. To receive student/resident rate, orders must be accompanied by name of affiliated institution, date of term, and the *signature* of program/ residency coordinator on institution letterhead. Orders will be billed at individual rate until proof of status received. Foreign air speed delivery is included in all *Clinics* subscription prices. All prices are subject to change without notice. **POSTMASTER:** Send address changes to *Rheumatic Disease Clinics of North America,* Elsevier Health Sciences Division, Subscription Customer Service, 3251 Riverport Lane, Maryland Heights, MO 63043. **Customer Service: 1-800-654-2452 (US and Canada). From outside of the US and Canada: 314-447-8871. Fax: 314-447-8029. For print support, e-mail: JournalsCustomerService-usa@elsevier.com. For online support, e-mail: JournalsOnlineSupport-usa@elsevier.com.**

Reprints. For copies of 100 or more of articles in this publication, please contact the Commercial Reprints Department, Elsevier Inc., 360 Park Avenue South, New York, New York, 10010-1710; Tel.: +1-212-633-3874, Fax: +1-212-633-3820, and E-mail: reprints@elsevier.com.

Rheumatic Disease Clinics of North America is covered in *MEDLINE/PubMed (Index Medicus), Current Contents/Clinical Medicine, Science Citation Index, ISI/BIOMED,* and *EMBASE/Excerpta Medica.*

Contributors

CONSULTING EDITOR

MICHAEL H. WEISMAN, MD
Distinguished Professor of Medicine Emeritus, David Geffen School of Medicine at UCLA, Professor of Medicine Emeritus, Cedars-Sinai Medical Center, Los Angeles, California

EDITORS

KARINA D. TORRALBA, MD, MACM, RhMSUS,
CCD, Chief and Fellowship Program Director, Professor of Medicine, Division of Rheumatology, Department of Medicine, Loma Linda University School of Medicine, Loma Linda, California

JAMES D. KATZ, MD
Senior Research Physician, Director, NIAMS Rheumatology Fellowship and Training Branch, Program Director, Rheumatology Fellowship, National Institutes of Health/NIAMS, Bethesda, Maryland

AUTHORS

JULIET AIZER, MD, MPH
Assistant Professor of Clinical Medicine, Nanette Laitman Education Scholar in Entrepreneurship, Assistant Attending Physician, Rheumatology, Weill Cornell Medicine, Hospital for Special Surgery, New York, New York

NEVENA BARJAKTAROVIC, MD
Rheumatology Fellow, Department of Medicine - Rheumatology, Albert Einstein College of Medicine, Bronx, New York

ANDREA M. BARKER, MPAS, PA-C
Adjunct Instructor, Department of Family and Preventive Medicine, Primary Care and Co-Director, Center of Excellence in Musculoskeletal Care and Education, George E. Wahlen VA Salt Lake City Health Care System, University of Utah Health Sciences Center, Salt Lake City VA Medical Center, Salt Lake City, Utah

MICHAEL J. BATTISTONE, MD
Associate Professor, Division of Rheumatology, Department of Medicine, Staff Physician and Director, Center of Excellence in Musculoskeletal Care and Education, George E. Wahlen VA Salt Lake City Health Care System, University of Utah Health Sciences Center, Salt Lake City VA Medical Center, Salt Lake City, Utah

IRENE BLANCO, MD, MS
Associate Professor of Medicine, Rheumatology Fellowship Program Director, Associate Dean of Diversity Enhancement, Department of Medicine - Rheumatology, Albert Einstein College of Medicine, Bronx, New York

AMY CANNELLA, MD, MS, RhMSUS
Associate Professor, UNMC Rheumatology, Nebraska Medical Center, Omaha VA Medical Center, Omaha, Nebraska

LISA CRISCIONE-SCHREIBER, MD, MEd
Fellowship Program Director, Division of Rheumatology and Immunology, Chair, Program for Women in Internal Medicine, Associate Vice Chair for Faculty Development and Diversity, Department of Medicine, Duke University School of Medicine, Durham, North Carolina

MEGAN L. CURRAN, MD
Associate Professor of Pediatrics, Section of Rheumatology, Children's Hospital of Colorado, University of Colorado School of Medicine, Aurora, Colorado

LOOMEE DOO, MD
Fellow, Division of Rheumatology, Department of Medicine, Loma Linda University Medical Center, Loma Linda, California

CHRISTINA DOWNEY, MD, RhMSUS
Assistant Professor of Medicine, Division of Rheumatology, Loma Linda University Medical Center, Loma Linda, California

STEVEN J. DURNING, MD, PhD, FACP
Professor of Medicine and Pathology, Staff Internist, Director, Graduate Programs in Health Professions Education, Uniformed Services University of the Health Sciences, Bethesda, Maryland

CANDACE H. FELDMAN, MD, MPH, ScD
Department of Medicine, Division of Rheumatology, Inflammation and Immunity, Brigham and Women's Hospital, Boston, Massachusetts

MARIANNA B. FREY, BA
Research Assistant, Rheumatology, Hospital for Special Surgery, New York, New York

CRISTINA M. GONZALEZ, MD, MEd
Associate Professor of Medicine, Attending Hospitalist, Department of Medicine - Hospital Medicine, Albert Einstein College of Medicine, Montefiore Medical Center, Bronx, New York

KRISTEN HAYWARD, MD, MS
Associate Professor of Pediatrics, Division of Rheumatology, Seattle Children's Hospital, University of Washington, School of Medicine, Seattle, Washington

DONNA M. JOSE, MD
Department of Internal Medicine, Loma Linda University, Loma Linda, California

JANE S. KANG, MD, MS
Associate Professor of Medicine, Fellowship Program Director, Division of Rheumatology, Columbia University Irving Medical Center, New York, New York

EUGENE Y. KISSIN, MD, RhMSUS
Associate Professor, Division of Rheumatology, Boston University Medical Center, Boston, Massachusetts

LISA A. MANDL, MD, MPH
Assistant Attending Physician, Rheumatology, Assistant Research Professor of Medicine and Assistant Research Professor of Healthcare Policy and Research, Weill Cornell Medicine, Hospital for Special Surgery, New York, New York

LINETT MARTIROSSIAN, MD
Rheumatology Fellow, Division of Rheumatology, Boston University Medical Center, Boston, Massachusetts

JAY MEHTA, MD, MSEd
Associate Professor of Clinical Pediatrics, Perelman School of Medicine, University of Pennsylvania, Children's Hospital of Philadelphia, Philadelphia, Pennsylvania

ELI M. MILOSLAVSKY, MD
Assistant Professor of Medicine, Division of Rheumatology, Allergy and Immunology, Department of Medicine, Massachusetts General Hospital, Harvard Medical School, Boston, Massachusetts

DEEPA RAGESH PANIKKATH, MD
Division of Rheumatology, Loma Linda University Medical Center, Loma Linda, California

REBECCA E. SADUN, MD, PhD
Assistant Professor of Medicine and Pediatrics, Adult and Pediatric Rheumatology, Duke University Medical Center, Durham, North Carolina

VANEET K. SANDHU, MD
Assistant Professor, Department of Internal Medicine, Division of Rheumatology, Loma Linda University, Loma Linda University Medical Center, Loma Linda, California

JULIE A. SCHELL, EdD, MS, BS
Executive Director for Extended and Executive Education, Assistant Professor of Practice, School of Design and Creative Technologies, College of Education, Dual Appointment, The University of Texas at Austin, Austin, Texas; Associate with Mazur Group, John A. Paulson School of Engineering and Applied Sciences, Harvard University, Cambridge, Massachusetts

NAOMI SERLING-BOYD, MD
Rheumatology Fellow, Division of Rheumatology, Allergy and Immunology, Department of Medicine, Massachusetts General Hospital, Harvard Medical School, Boston, Massachusetts

DANIEL H. SOLOMON, MD, MPH
Divisions of Rheumatology, Immunology and Allergy and Pharmacoepidemiology, Brigham and Women's Hospital, Harvard Medical School, Boston, Massachusetts

MICHAEL D. TIONGSON, BA
Medical Student, Albany Medical College, Albany, New York

KARINA D. TORRALBA, MD, MACM, RhMSUS
CCD, Chief and Fellowship Program Director, Professor of Medicine, Division of Rheumatology, Department of Medicine, Loma Linda University School of Medicine, Loma Linda, California

BENJAMIN B. WIDENER, MD
UNMC Rheumatology Fellow, Nebraska Medical Center, Omaha VA Medical Center, Omaha, Nebraska

Contents

Lectures, a form of passive learning, are a modality of teaching used in medical education. Active learning strategies allow learners and teachers to interact and be more engaged with the subject matter in a manner that encourages discussion, critical thinking, and advanced clinical reasoning skills. Learning to be effective requires vigilance, which promotes memory retention and should afford a way for learners to build on preexisting knowledge via scaffolding and concept mapping that uses critical thinking. Educators should also to use evaluation models that seek to improve patient care, health care systems, and community health.

Objective structured clinical examinations assess learners "showing how" to perform complex clinical tasks. Devised as summative evaluations, these examinations with immediate feedback are useful formative evaluations to improve learner performance. This review describes how objective structured clinical examinations have been used in rheumatology education. Steps for creating an objective structured clinical examination are discussed. Validity and reproducibility are important considerations, especially for high-stakes summative objective structured clinical examinations. Consideration of the potential benefits in clinical education and their hazards are reviewed. When well-designed, formative objective structured clinical examinations have high educational value for learners and medical educators.

"E-learning" refers to instruction occurring via digital media and ideally uses an engaging and learner-centered approach. Advantages of e-learning methods include (1) they can enable consistent messages, (2) they may use novel instructional methods, and (3) they enable documentation of usage and assessment. This article discusses principles for and challenges to developing e-learning materials. The authors provide a collection of available e-learning materials used to teach adult and pediatric rheumatology developed by individuals, professional societies, and private companies. Finally, they discuss challenges to using e-learning materials.

Ultrasound in rheumatology is gaining increasing acceptance in the field, with its use expanding beyond the musculoskeletal system to image rheumatic disease pathology of the vasculature, salivary glands, and lungs. Fellows in training and practicing clinicians are seeking ways to attain training and competency assessment. These standards are evolving, but no uniform mechanism for training exists. Although clinicians in practice find a wide array of resources available for self-directed education in ultrasound in rheumatology, a consensus-based and publicly available training curriculum can further enhance and standardize learning. This article discusses ultrasound in rheumatology education opportunities, competency assessment, and certification pathways.

Subspecialty consultation is an increasingly used resource in inpatient medicine. Teaching the primary team is an important element of effective consultation and has many potential benefits. However, within academic medical centers many barriers to effective consultation and the consult learning environment exist. High workload, burnout, inexperience, lack of familiarity between teams, quality of the consult requests, and pushback may impede teaching and learning. Herein, the authors review the role of teaching and learning during consultation, challenges to effective consultation facing fellows, and interventions that can enhance primary team-fellow interactions and learning.

 Video content accompanies this article at http://www.rheumatic. theclinics.com.

To provide optimal patient care, rheumatologists must be equipped and motivated to critically appraise the literature. The conceptual frameworks Retrieval Enhanced Learning, Self-Determination Theory, and Communities of Practice can inform the design of educational approaches to promote critical appraisal in practice. HSS CLASS-Rheum® is a learning tool that can be used to help rheumatologists learn skills for critical appraisal through retrieval practice. Combining retrieval practice with opportunities for connection through Peer Instruction, journal clubs, and other forums can help support engagement and internalization of motivation, promoting persistence with critical appraisal in practice.

Adolescence and young adulthood represents a vulnerable period in the life of patients with rheumatic diseases, many of whom struggle with chronic disease self-management and with adjustment to adult rheumatology care. Often, adult rheumatologists are uncomfortable caring for young adults, especially those with pediatric-onset diagnoses. The recent development of evidence-based best practices, expert opinion recommendations, and validated tools can assist pediatric and adult rheumatologists in caring for adolescent and young adult patients. Uptake of these guidelines and resources remains low, however, underscoring the need for rheumatologists and trainees to receive explicit training in the application of transition best practices.

Physicians in training and their mentors must be cognizant of ethical concerns related to industry interactions. Mentors perceived to have conflicts of interest or to be engaging in misconduct can unconsciously and profoundly affect the learning and academic environment by implying certain values and expectations. Despite increased awareness of ethical concerns related to industry interactions in clinical practice and research, there remains a need for interventions to prevent ethical transgressions. Ethics education is essential and a move in the right direction, but it alone is likely inadequate in preventing unethical behavior. Education should be supplemented with ethical environments at institutions.

This article reviews several national programs in musculoskeletal education initiated by the Department of Veterans Affairs over the past decade. These programs have become sustained interprofessional opportunities for learners across disciplines and along the continuum of health professions education (HPE) and training pathways. This article also describes opportunities for leaders in rheumatology and other HPE programs to join these efforts and to collaborate in the scholarship that will be necessary in constructing educational programs fit for the purpose of ensuring a well-trained, competent workforce of health care providers.

Academic institutions play an essential role in providing physicians with the necessary skills needed to improve the quality and value of care provided. The Accreditation Council for Graduate Medical Education has several milestones in the curriculum of fellowship programs that prioritize involvement in quality improvement (QI) and patient safety efforts. This article reviews the unique benefits and challenges of involving and teaching fellows to conduct QI initiatives. Strategies and resources available to overcome these challenges and develop a successful quality driven training environment are outlined in this article.

The shortage of health care professionals is projected to worsen in the coming years. This is particularly concerning in underserved areas that are fraught with disparities in disease outcomes and life expectancy, quality of life, and health care access. The onus is on medical education institutions to train students to serve vulnerable communities to improve both health care access and the quality of medical school education. When health disparities are formally included in medical education curricula and the culture of medical education shifts to a community-based learning approach, patients and health care providers alike will reap the benefits.

Health and health care disparities are present in every medical specialty, and stem from multiple etiologies. Within health care itself, issues mostly arise within medical providers and across a system with an inequitable distribution of care and resources. One potential way to address disparities is to educate our workforce, to not only know about disparities but to also actively advocate for underresourced and marginalized patients. In this review, the authors describe efforts being conducted in graduate medical education and seek to elucidate some of the curricula currently being developed and implemented in rheumatology.

RHEUMATIC DISEASE CLINICS OF NORTH AMERICA

FORTHCOMING ISSUES

May 2020
Spondyloarthritis: The Changing Landscape Today
Xenofon Baraliakos and
Michael Weisman, *Editors*

August 2020
Cancer and Rheumatic Diseases
John Davis, *Editor*

November 2020
Health Disparities in Rheumatic Diseases
Candace H. Feldman, *Editor*

RECENT ISSUES

November 2019
Treat to Target in Rheumatic Diseases: Rationale and Results
Daniel Aletaha, *Editor*

August 2019
Controversies in Rheumatology
Jonathan Kay and Sergio Schwartzman, *Editors*

May 2019
Technology and Big Data in Rheumatology
Jeffrey R. Curtis, Kaleb Michaud, and Kevin Winthrop, *Editors*

SERIES OF RELATED INTEREST

Medical Clinics of North America
https://www.medical.theclinics.com/
Neurologic Clinics
https://www.neurologic.theclinics.com/
Dermatologic Clinics
https://www.derm.theclinics.com/
Physical Medicine and Rehabilitation Clinics of North America
https://www.pmr.theclinics.com/

THE CLINICS ARE AVAILABLE ONLINE!
Access your subscription at:
www.theclinics.com

Foreword

Education and Professional Development in Rheumatology

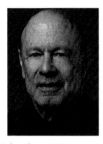

Michael H. Weisman, MD
Consulting Editor

The genesis of this issue is critical to our understanding of its impact. Jim Katz contacted the series editor some time ago to suggest that the *Rheumatic Disease Clinics of North America* take the lead as a resource for scientific contributions for the topic of graduate medical education in rheumatology. After some discussions about how to do this, we landed on an issue that not only addresses education but also is broad enough to include professional development. We explicitly requested, and now we have, a deliverable well beyond our expectations, that it be scholarly, credible, and academically sound. Clearly, the clinician-educators have come of age, and this issue has exceeded our initial goals. We are especially proud of Jim and Karina for doing this.

Torralba and Doo deliver a remarkable article on how to improve medical education by employing active learning strategies that translate into critical thinking and actionable experiences for the learner. They clearly address how to take preexisting knowledge and integrate it into the learner's ability to engage the subject matter. This article is a must-read for anyone who thinks they want to be a clinician-educator.

The evolution of objective structured clinical examinations as educational tools has reached a high point for Rheumatology, and Lisa Criscione-Schreiber does a remarkable job in describing the high educational value of these activities.

Megan Curran discusses the risks and benefits of "e-learning" and the impact of such activities as challenges for all stakeholders in the educational field.

Widener and colleagues discuss the expanding use of ultrasound beyond the musculoskeletal system, but they also sound the alarm for the need to develop standardized and accepted methods of competency assessment.

Serling-Boyd and Miloslavsky address the complex and often talked about, but never studied seriously, teaching experience in the in-patient consultation setting. Workload, burnout, and other barriers to effective communication need research attention.

Rheum Dis Clin N Am 46 (2020) xiii–xiv
https://doi.org/10.1016/j.rdc.2019.10.002
0889-857X/20/© 2019 Published by Elsevier Inc.

rheumatic.theclinics.com

Aizer and associates introduce us to an often-forgotten piece of education: how to critically appraise the literature. Her colleagues at Hospital for Special Surgery have developed a tool to help in this regard, but they also recognize the need to internalize these steps to sustain the activity when the Fellows leave the institutional environment.

Rebecca Sadun identifies young adulthood as a particularly vulnerable period for our patients with rheumatic diseases; based on adult learning theory, she has given us excellent suggestions to enhance the learning experience of our Fellows as they approach this challenge.

Jane Kang does a beautiful job in discussing the ethical issues facing our relationships to pharmaceutical companies, but she goes beyond the basics and tells us that the entire ethical atmosphere at each institution has a profound effect on what people will actually do going forward.

Battistone and colleagues, from the vantage point of the Veterans Administration health care system, have developed creative methods to enhance the skills of primary care providers as well as health professional education students. They share them with us.

Downey and colleagues teach us how to implement Quality Improvement projects within the education of our Fellows: this is an important and essential piece of our training environment.

Sandhu and colleagues address the educational challenges posed by our vulnerable communities and the need to implement community-based learning approaches that benefit all concerned.

Finally, Blanco and colleagues drill down on health care disparities in today's world of inequitable distribution of resources. They describe curricula currently being developed that address this gap in the education of our Fellows, perhaps to encourage them in the long run to advocate for changes in the health care environment that benefit our patients.

Michael H. Weisman, MD
David Geffen School of Medicine at UCLA
Cedars-Sinai Medical Center
1545 Calmar Court
Los Angeles, CA 90024, USA

E-mail address:
Michael.Weisman@cshs.org

Preface

From Knowledge to Action: A Modern Venture in Rheumatology Education

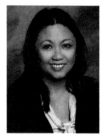 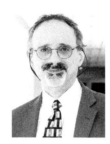

Karina D. Torralba, MD, MACM, RhMSUS   James D. Katz, MD
Editors

Apprenticeship embodies the traditional approach to medical education. Impactful learning moments during apprenticeship-style training may be brief and on-the-fly, or structured and proscribed. As an immediate and immersive experience, apprenticeship ensures supervised progress from "observership" status to legitimate peripheral participation, and then ultimately to clinical independence. To this end, graduate medical education (GME) is more than didactics. It encompasses feedback, assessment, and simulation training. At its core is the fundamental process of developing a trusting working-learning relationship between mentor and trainee as well as cultivating a nurturing learning environment. This demands higher sophistication with regard to the clinician's teaching skill set and a program director's ability to mitigate and mediate adverse factors in the environment.

Accreditation is an industry that drives modern GME. It has identified poor formal training of clinician-educators (so called "doctor-teachers") as a vulnerability that is deserving of more oversight. For example, incorporating training in the areas of patient safety, hospital governance, provider burnout, and ethics is a learning objective at the forefront of modern training programs. This emphasis recognizes the fact that doctors are increasingly being asked to take on socially critical roles, such as being advocates for their patients in a complex health system, innovating in health care delivery, and leading in both policy and interprofessional collaboration. Traditionally, these enumerated objectives reflect gaps in the education of trainees. Curriculum development aiming at redressing such gaps heavily relies upon adult learning theory. Ultimately, improving patient care and the GME clinical learning environment is the goal. It is therefore our earnest hope that this issue of *Rheumatic Disease Clinics of North America* furthers the art of teaching so as to embrace the various roles doctors are expected to

Rheum Dis Clin N Am 46 (2020) xv–xvi
https://doi.org/10.1016/j.rdc.2019.10.001
0889-857X/20/© 2019 Published by Elsevier Inc.

rheumatic.theclinics.com

fulfill while at the same time moving rheumatology education forward from knowledge to relevant action.

Karina D. Torralba, MD, MACM, RhMSUS
Division of Rheumatology
Department of Medicine
Loma Linda University
School of Medicine
11234 Anderson Street, MC 1519
Loma Linda, CA 92373, USA

James D. Katz, MD
National Institutes of Health/NIAMS
10N-311A
Building 10
9000 Rockville Pike
Bethesda, MD 20892, USA

E-mail addresses:
ktorralba@llu.edu (K.D. Torralba)
james.katz@nih.gov (J.D. Katz)

Active Learning Strategies to Improve Progression from Knowledge to Action

Karina D. Torralba, MD, MACM[a],*, Loomee Doo, MD[b]

KEYWORDS

- Rheumatology • Active learning • Musculoskeletal disease • Arthritis
- Concept mapping • Medical education

KEY POINTS

- Active learning presents an opportunity for both learners and teachers to interact and be more engaged with the subject matter in a manner that encourages discussion and critical thinking, and to build on preexisting knowledge using scaffolding and concept mapping skills.
- Lectures, a form of passive learning, carry the risk of mind wandering, leading to a decrement in learning vigilance.
- There are various strategies of active learning, including ways that also intersperse with the more effective use of lectures to relay information.
- It is important for educators to be cognizant of the various models of learning, frameworks for setting objectives, assessing competence, clinical problem-solving skills, and outcomes of learning when planning and carrying out their teaching strategy.
- Several studies by rheumatology educators have been done that have effectively assessed the use of various learning strategies for both undergraduate and postgraduate medical education.

EDUCATIONAL CONUNDRUMS

What is the best way to learn? What is the best way to teach? Knowledge is power, because knowledge is expected to lead to action. It is therefore imperative that how clinicians teach harnesses this empowerment to action. A couple of cases are presented to emphasize this point.

Disclosure: Regarding the team-based learning project described in this article, funding for this project was provided by the Rheumatology Research Foundation Clinician Scholar Educator Award. The authors have no other disclosures.
^a Division of Rheumatology, Department of Medicine, Loma Linda University School of Medicine, 11234 Anderson Street, MC 1519, Loma Linda, CA 92373, USA; ^b Division of Rheumatology, Department of Medicine, Loma Linda University Medical Center, Loma Linda, CA, USA
* Corresponding author.
E-mail address: ktorralba@llu.edu

Rheum Dis Clin N Am 46 (2020) 1–19
https://doi.org/10.1016/j.rdc.2019.09.001
0889-857X/20/© 2019 Elsevier Inc. All rights reserved.

rheumatic.theclinics.com

Case 1: Conference blues

A rheumatologist in the clinician-educator track is tasked to teach 100 residents for a 1-hour noontime core curriculum session on the topic of management of rheumatoid arthritis. She determines that, after this session, she wants each resident to know how to make a diagnosis of rheumatoid arthritis, and to initiate initial treatment of rheumatoid arthritis.

Problem: She highly doubts that giving a 60-minute lecture is the best way to keep the residents' attention sustained, or the best way to determine whether the residents will understand her teaching points.

Case 2: When a fracture portends a future fracture

Rheumatology received a consult from orthopedic surgery regarding a 55-year old woman for management of her lupus and osteoporosis. The patient sustained a right intertrochanteric fracture sustained after a ground-level fall. Two years ago, she had a left hip fracture. For her lupus, she has been on prednisone 7.5 mg daily for the past 10 years. She has not had dual-energy X-ray absorptiometry, has not been on calcium and vitamin D supplementation, nor prophylaxis or treatment of osteoporosis.

Problem: the orthopedic surgery physician and resident relate that it is common for them to have patients coming in for repeat fragility fractures without osteoporosis treatment having been initiated. A medical literature and electronic medical record review for fragility fracture hospitalizations for the past 12 months shows that an osteoporosis care gap exists, and that 60% of patients coming in with a fracture had a prior fracture. The attendings and trainees agree not only to a joint morbidity and mortality conference but also to a collaborative venture to enact systems change to prevent more fractures.

INTRODUCTION

Physicians are defined not only by the medical knowledge they possess and the patient care they provide but also by the roles and characteristics that enable them to (1) stay current with the ever-changing science and technology; (2) be socially responsible; and (3) affect systems change to ensure patient safety, quality of care, and community health.[1–4] These roles require analysis and synthesis of problems, creation and application of solutions, and evaluation tools to determine the effectiveness of these solutions.[5–8] It therefore becomes imperative for educators to teach in a manner that embraces development of these skill sets in the form of active learning strategies.[9,10]

Active learning is a learner-centered learning method involving active participation whether through reading, writing, or discussion in class. In contrast with lectures, in which learners passively listen to teachers, rarely ask questions, and are summatively assessed during a test at a future date, active learners are participants who are expected to prepare for class discussions in advance and develop thought-provoking, relevant questions that encourage dialogue and collaborative learning in the classroom setting. Here, the teacher is no longer viewed as a pedagogical figure who bestows knowledge to students but instead as a facilitator that nurtures conversation in the classroom[11–15] (**Table 1**). Passive learning through traditional lectures is still the teaching strategy predominantly used in medical education, whether in the medical school, postgraduate medical education, or professional continuing medical education levels. Although valued as a teaching strategy to deliver important and concise information, lectures by themselves are ill-equipped to provide deep formative learning, which is characterized by active learning, critical thinking, and clinical reasoning.[10]

Table 1
Key differences between passive lecture-based learning versus active learning

	Passive Learning	Active Learning
Forms/Examples	Traditional lecture	Problem-based learning, team-based learning
Teacher Role	Imparts information, subject expert usually	Facilitates discussion, may or may not be subject expert
Student Role	Imbibes information	Engages in discourse and other activities, asks questions, researches answers
Interpersonal Skills, Teamwork	Minimal opportunities; students are passive listeners while teachers lecture	High; activities are designed to engage teachers with learners, and learners between themselves
Critical Thinking	Minimal; learners may learn material and largely self-determine clinical thinking and reasoning skills without guidance by teacher	High; activities are designed to engage students toward a higher level of understanding of the subject matter
Accountability	Tests developed by teachers are used to check student learning	Onus is on learners to drive discussions and determine depth of knowledge. Learners need to be prepared for teaching sessions and to participate in activities

The Flipped Classroom Can Be Anywhere

Active learning has been closely aligned with the term flipped classroom (2012). This term has gained popularity because learners are expected to equip themselves with base knowledge before the class (which may be in the form of reading materials or recorded lectures), and then do the homework in class through engagement with activities that encourage investigation, complex thinking, and peer-peer or peer-teacher interaction. In this manner, the learner must activate newly gained knowledge and evaluate whether the information makes sense.[11] Learners may be asked to assess the validity of given literature by delving into more recent literature that can either support or refute what is taught in the classroom. Learners also develop communication skills by debating their thoughts and articulating their opinions during discussions. These skills will help students to become better thinkers, reinforce knowledge, and create a foundation to become future teachers. In Brazil, active learning was tested on 72 residents to determine whether ward teaching is more effective by active learning versus traditional teaching. Active learning resulted in improved knowledge acquisition at least three times more compared with traditional learning.[16]

It should be emphasized that active learning does not only occur in classroom settings, which are typically associated with the lecture hall format, but may apply to any session in which didactics and any other exchange of information are involved, including conferences done as part of postgraduate medical training. The Accreditation Council of Graduate Medical Education (ACGME) requires didactic sessions or conferences during rheumatology training (particularly clinical case, research, morbidity and mortality, and quality improvement conferences), to be done in a manner that requires interaction between peers and among peer and faculty.[17]

Educational Psychology and Theory Behind Active Learning

Learning requires mindful vigilance

For learning to be effective, regardless of the form, the learner is required to have a certain level of attentional state. Mind wandering (ie, daydreaming, zoning out, tuning out) tends to occur among learners listening to lectures.[18] The longer a lecture is, the higher the inability to sustain this attentional state (vigilance decrement), decreasing the chances of memory retention.[18,19] This prompts questions of how long is too long, and whether boring speakers talk for longer. An attempt to answer these questions was made in a small study in a single setting in which a series of 12-minute talks were judged by the author functioning as the determiner of the degree of boredom. The difference between a boring talk versus an interesting talk was about 90 seconds (11 minutes, 42 seconds vs 13 minutes, 12 seconds); every 70 seconds that a speaker continued talking, the odds that the talk had become boring doubled.[20]

Building on preexisting learned knowledge

There are several theories of adult learning that lend to active learning. Active learning has 4 key requirements: activating prior knowledge; involving most of the students; promoting student metacognition, including reflection; providing students with feedback about their learning.[11] Scaffolding, which is the structural process by which teachers provider learners, progressive understanding of content towards independent learning, is particularly important in medicine in which the content can be complex and overly abundant.[10] However, for learning to be meaningful, this depends on learners having a preexisting base of knowledge to build on. Building this scaffold requires critical thinking and reasoning whereby learners choose to assimilate further information by being able to think of concepts related to base knowledge. This process is fully described by Joseph Novak's[21] theory of education, known as human constructivism, which in turn is based on the Ausubel assimilation theory. This approach to learning is exemplified by creation of a concept map wherein learners can designate relationships between new information and preexisting knowledge based on their evaluation and understanding of the information received.[22] Operationally, learning processes can be described in the context of Bloom[5] taxonomy (and further revisions by Anderson and colleagues[6]), and the Miller[7] pyramid. The process of evaluation of learning and its outcomes is also vital and this is elucidated by the Fitzpatrick model.[8] Although there is no complete correlation with each as to how they fit with one another, the side-by-side schema presented in (**Fig. 1**) provides some foundation for clinician educators to begin to understand these various concepts and how they relate to one another.

Processes of concept mapping can be harnessed for use in active learning.[23,24] Concept mapping that derives from illness scripts can delineate a process of clinical reasoning skills development.[25–27] Novice learners, such as medical students or early first-year residents, may have an understanding of basic pathophysiology, clinical correlation, and the initial management of common illnesses. These concepts become ingrained with repetition and reflection. However, higher-level learning characterized by refined discrimination of clinical features and the application of more sophisticated reasoning skills to complex scenarios is the goal of active learning (**Fig. 2**). The Dreyfus model of clinician problem-solving skills illustrates how learners evolve from being novice learners, who are knowledgeable about the pathophysiology and management of common and simple conditions, to experts, who are able to build reliably on prior knowledge to be able to make higher-level decisions for more complex or even rare conditions. The Dreyfus model actually serves as the framework for the ACGME

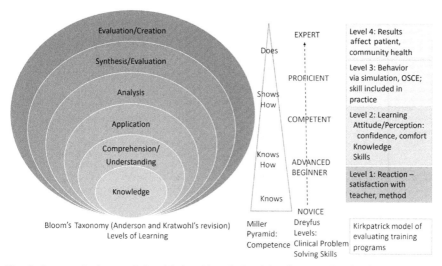

Fig. 1. Proposed schema of the side-by-side relationship of various levels of learning with levels of competence (Miller pyramid), ability to achieve clinical problem-solving skills (Dreyfus levels), and evaluation outcomes (Kirkpatrick and Kirkpatrick framework). OSCE, objective structured clinical examination.

Milestones which are explicitly defined and evaluable trainee knowledge, skills, behaviors, and performance outcomes for each of the competencies.[17] These serve as a trajectory for trainees in postgraduate medical education to achieve competence, and for educators to be able to evaluate a trainees' achievement of expertise.

Advantages of Active Learning

There are tangible advantages to active learning.[12,28]

Building and questioning

Students learn communication skills by developing ways to debate their thoughts and articulate their opinions during active learning discussions. They learn to build on preexisting knowledge, get the opportunity to question preconceived notions, test hypotheses, and develop new concepts. These skills help students to become better thinkers, reinforce their knowledge, and create a foundation to become future teachers.

Teachers do more than teach

For teachers used to giving lectures, active learning can be a learning opportunity in several ways: (1) to expand their teaching skills; (2) to learn new insights from learners themselves; (3) to receive immediate feedback at the time of their engagement with the learner to assess whether their teaching technique is effective or too esoteric, which they can adjust by providing additional or alternative explanations; and (4) to engage with learners at a more personal level by being motivators and listeners themselves. It requires a different method of preparation: instead of merely preparing slides or notes to assist with discourse, the preparation entails allotment of time, materials, and methods to incorporate active learning, regardless of which form of active learning is used. Teaching becomes a dialogue and can foster a relationship among students and teachers that can develop into mentorship.

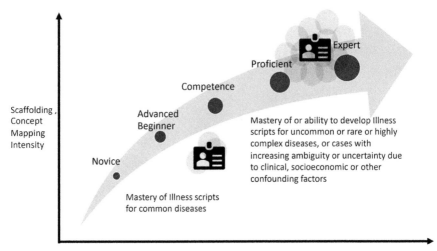

Dreyfus Levels of clinician problem-solving skills

Fig. 2. Relationship between level of problem-solving skills by a clinician (Dreyfus levels) and ability to build up on preexisting knowledge using scaffolding and concept mapping. Icon with person and notes denotes an illness script. Each circle symbolizes a nidus of knowledge; where they are more circles, there is increasing knowledge, an expansion of a scaffold. Grayness denotes ambiguity.

Active Learning Takes Many Forms

Active learning has evolved to include multiple teaching styles that can cater to different subjects and student populations (see **Table 1**). Active learning does not mean it is devoid of lectures, but instead lectures can be used in more effective ways as a means to relay information in combination with other strategies that reinforce learning. Active learning can also be categorized according to learning theory pedagogy: constructivism, problem-based learning (PBL), discovery-based learning, inquiry-based learning, and project-based learning.[29] Regardless of which pedagogy is entertained, all forms are learner centered. Although detailed discussion of each form of active learning, including their advantages and disadvantages, is beyond the scope of this article, some key studies are highlighted that have used active learning techniques in rheumatology[30–41] (see **Table 3**). Articles were selected if they gave explicit information regarding using case-based learning (CBL), team-based learning (TBL), PBL, or other interactive in-person strategies, including how they assessed the effectiveness of their interventions. Active learning can also be done on an individual basis, such as through the use of interactive Web-based modules,[42] and through interprofessional collaborative venues[43]; however, these are described in other articles in this issue.

Although **Table 2** elaborates on many active learning techniques used in various rheumatology curricula, some of these studies included active learning in combination with other teaching strategies. Only a few[31,32,36,41] used specific active learning techniques that showed outcomes directly affecting patient health. Guillen-Astete and colleagues[36] were able to show the achievement of advanced-level outcomes of learning related to changes in behavior or practice most likely caused by the specificity of covered topics, in this case back pain, which makes measuring of adoption of such knowledge and skills and linking this to the effects of the educational intervention more feasible.

Table 2
Forms of active learning

Types of Active Learning	Definition
Pause for reflection/ "muddiest" point[13]	• Take a few minutes to reflect on what you learned that day • What part was the most difficult or unclear (muddiest) then discuss soon after
Think, pair, share[11]	• Idea/thought is given by instructor • Students have individual time to reflect • Students are paired up to share ideas • Pairs are joined in larger groups to discuss ideas
Harvesting[13]	• Soon after a topic is discussed, instructor asks 2 questions: • "So what?" (ie, why is this important?) • "Now what?" (what will you do with this information?) • Allows learners to take away the meaningfulness behind the teaching and instructors learn their students' level of understanding
Figure analysis[14]	• Similar to think-pair-share in the science classroom • Figures are shown and individuals analyze them • Share the figures, interpret the meaning in pairs • Regroup in a large discussion to discuss the figures, critically think, and analyze the results expressed in the figures
Peer review[12]	• Large group divides into small groups and select a research topic to write an article/present • Each small group exchanges drafts and gives feedback • Then instructor evaluate drafts before groups present final products
PBL/case studies[11]	• Students read about case studies and engage in a large group discussion on certain questions posed in the studies • Led by instructor guidance
Brainstorming/ "fishbone"[12]	• A large group is separated into smaller groups • Each group takes a "bone," or factor that affects the overall outcome ("fish"), and take 5–10 min to discuss in small groups • The groups reconvene in a larger discussion and take turns sharing their perspectives on how their bone affects the overall fish
Hands-on technology[11]	• Use audience response systems (clickers) for student participation in PowerPoint presentations
Active review sessions (games/ simulations)[12]	• Instructor prepares a game, such as jeopardy, for student groups to compete and answer • Simulations of situations such as cardiopulmonary resuscitation, intubations, and line placements are demonstrated. The students then participate in simulations and regroup afterward to discuss what they have learned as well as the challenges and receive feedback
Role playing/ "thinking hats"[13]	• Students prepare and perform a skit to illustrate a concept • Classmates play different roles in a dialogue prepared by the teacher • Encourages critical thinking, identifies root causes and factors that can affect outcomes
Jigsaw discussion[12]	• Large group is divided into small groups (ie, group A, B, and C) to discuss a topic • Then 1 member of each group joins with 1 member of the other groups (ie, A + B + C = 1 team) and teaches each other what they have learned

(*continued on next page*)

Table 2 (continued)	
Types of Active Learning	**Definition**
Experiential learning (site visits)[12]	• Students take field trips to sites to experience what they have learned in the classroom (eg, going to nursing homes in geriatrics, visiting museums for art class, aquariums for biology)
Forum theater[15]	• Used in moral education classrooms • Script: a script is developed showing a moral conflict • Antimodel: the script is performed by actors in which they succumb to this moral conflict • Forum: another instructor discusses the problems with the situation and possible solutions • Intervention play: play is restarted but paused and intervened by audience members until the conflict is resolved

Problem-Based Learning

One of the most popular teaching methods using active learning in large group settings is PBL. Commonly PBL is structured with students assigned to specific roles and then working in teams. A facilitator who is a group process expert and a facilitator with medical expertise is assigned to each team. The teacher facilitates the discussion on a problem and all participants express their hypotheses and theories as to the root of the problem as well as possible solutions. Then everyone individually researches the problem and regroups to present their findings. The goal of this technique is not to reach a preset conclusion but to promote collaboration among members and to create new meaning through reflection and reasoning.[44] As a result, team members learn to critically appraise ideas, support and guide one another, all the while emphasizing a mindset of lifelong learning. When introduced early in the education trajectory, students realize the importance of teamwork and develop the self-motivation and persistence to find answers that, it is hoped, will embed lifelong learning habits as they advance in their careers.

Team-Based Learning

TBL is also used for large group settings with learners grouped into teams. It varies from PBL in several ways: (1) it makes learners accountable for mastery of base material in advance of classroom sessions by requiring them to review materials (eg, video, prerecorded lecture, articles); (2) learners are required to prepare for activities to be done in class and are required to evaluate each other on their ability to work as a team. In essence, students assume the role of the teacher as a facilitator or instructor in lieu of the presence of a group process expert as would occur in PBL. Accountability is enabled by the TBL process because it involves completing an individual readiness assurance test (IRAT) followed by a group readiness assurance test (GRAT), ultimately followed by a case application.[45]

A modified TBL strategy was adopted by one of the authors (K.T.) for internal medicine resident noontime core curriculum learning sessions (CCLSs).[31,32] The objectives of the study were:

1. To determine the level of receptiveness of the residents to the TBL strategy
2. To determine their attitudes toward the importance of teamwork in learning and professional success

3. To determine whether the level of attendance is a determining factor in In-Training Exam (ITE) score achievement

Over 3 years, 18 TBL CCLSs participated in by postgraduate year 1 to 3 residents have been conducted. Two surveys administered after the session showed positive results: (1) a rheumatology TBL learning evaluation survey showed that the use of TBL allowed learners to interact and learn from the material, their colleagues, and the instructor, and showed that the objectives were well defined and that the activities were organized; (2) a Value of Teams© (Baylor College of Medicine) survey showed largely positive responses to the importance of teamwork and collaboration for successful student work and careers, whereas most of the responses were positive. The possible effect of TBL participation on ITE scores was assessed. Out of 129 interns and 2 residents, 13 had no record of attendance, 81 had a low level of attendance (1–4 sessions), and 35 had a medium level of attendance (5–9 sessions). Analysis of variance showed a significant difference in rheumatology ITE scores. Scheffe post hoc analysis showed that residents with a medium level of attendance had significantly higher rheumatology ITE scores compared with those that did not participate or had a low level of attendance. Overall, residents were receptive to TBL strategy for CCLSs. There was an overall positive response to valuing the importance of teams. Residents participating in 5 to 9 TBL sessions over a 2-year period were more likely to have significantly higher rheumatology ITE scores compared with those that did not participate or who participated in fewer than 5 sessions.

Yoong and Lui[46] discussed the changes they made to the rheumatology and immunology curricular interventions that they have used at the undergraduate and postgraduate Singapore General Hospital, including the use of information technologies.

Active Learning: Impact to Rheumatology Academic Educator Workforce

Barriers to active learning: the educator's dilemma

Active learning has its challenges. Most of the published studies on active learning are done at the medical school level, less so at the postgraduate training level, where conferences can be less structured, flexible, and easily disrupted because of competing clinical demands.[47,48]

Barriers included limitations set by conference rooms (size, table/chair setup); clinical work (pages/messages coming in); faculty training (lack of training, discomfort with a perception of losing control); and perception of, or lack of, learner buy-in (engagement).[47–49] Teachers new to active learning may be uncomfortable with the notion of being a facilitator and motivator: it takes a certain mixture of charisma and courage to transform into someone both engaging with and inspiring to the learners. Students not interested in the subject matter may be resistant to engaging in interactive activities. Students also may not want to work together. It takes a personality and mindset of open-mindedness on the part of both teacher and learner to successfully engage in active learning. The active learning activities may be time consuming, or alternatively might be perceived as being too chaotic. Identification of specific learning goals and objectives is key to a successful teaching session.

Adoption of active learning entails social risk. Because active learning in certain settings, such as TBL or PBL, encourages questioning authority, ambiguity and uncertainty associated with answering such questions may be uncomfortable for faculty and students alike, which may reflect ambiguity aversion and physicians' attitudes to communicating uncertainty.[50] It has been noted overall that successful active learning occurs when there is mutual effort and trust by both learners and faculty.[51]

Educator Faculty Workforce

Rheumatology faces an overall workforce shortage.[52] However, as of 2014, it no longer faces a rheumatology fellowship applicant shortage. Rheumatology fellowship application is now as competitive as cardiology, hematology, oncology, pulmonology, and gastroenterology. Instead, there exists a shortage of available rheumatology positions. Out of 358 applicants for 2018, 119 (33.2%) were unable to match to any program.[53]

Rheumatology clinician educators are a struggling subgroup. Goldenberg and colleagues[54] noted that rheumatologists in the early 1980s had limited involvement with medical school teaching or in instruction of the musculoskeletal examination. Furthermore, over the course of their training, the percentage of fellows wanting to go into an academic career (let alone clinician educator) decreases from 70% to 40% or less during the course of their fellowship. This decision may be influenced by financial considerations (eg, student loan repayment, lower faculty salaries) and lack of career development opportunities.[55] The use of a curriculum to equip fellows with teaching skills is promising for redressing this deficiency but whether or not this type of training affects the ultimate choice to pursue careers as clinician educators remains to be seen.[56]

Clinician-Educator Faculty Development

It therefore becomes imperative that clinician-educator faculty development should be a priority. However, recognition for this need and the provision of funding remain a problem.[57–59] An expanded educator's repertoire of teaching strategies is expected to better equip academic rheumatologists to confront the rapidly evolving field of graduate medical education. However, the competing demands on clinician-educator faculty present resource allocation challenges rendering the use of active learning strategies such as PBL problematic. PBL requires a large faculty commitment. Alternatively, TBL allows more efficient allocation of faculty resources; in TBL, 1 teacher (facilitator) can handle as many as 100 students grouped into 5 learners.[31,32] Self-directed learning is another approach designed to offload the burden on faculty time, including the use of existing electronic modules for preclass learner preparation.[42,60,61]

Faculty also need be equipped with knowledge and skills on how to develop teaching materials. For instance, faculty can use concept mapping as a means of planning teaching material, and as a teaching and assessment tool. Concept mapping allows educators and learners alike to visualize knowledge processes by organizing things by relationships to facilitate understanding.[62] Concept maps can be used as a pre-class, or in-class, activity; may be used as a way to summarize information; and can be used to assess learner understanding. If used in determining a patient's treatment plan, the concept map can be used, for example, to map a problem's possible solutions.[63] Concept mapping is just one of many techniques. A complete discussion of strategies for developing teaching materials is beyond the scope of this paper. A useful resource is the MedEdPortal which features peer-reviewed materials developed by educators, sponsored the Association of American Medical Colleges.[64]

In addition to teaching strategies, training is required in the assessment of learner outcomes. **Table 3** lists some of the assessments used to evaluate the effectiveness of active learning strategies. Objective structured clinical examination–related resources already developed by region-wide collaborations may be adopted. The use

Table 3
Rheumatology-specific curricula indicating use of specific active learning techniques

Author/Year/Location	Learner Population	Topics	Interventions	Assessments	Outcome (Fitzpatrick Model[b])
Scheers-Masters et al,[30] 2011[a] Brooklyn, NY	PGY1 neurology, medicine	Clinical experience/ diseases, arthrocentesis, and injection techniques	Case-based modules, quizzes, rotations, skills simulators, clinics, journal club	Multiple choice test, OSCE postquestionnaire	Knowledge, skills, attitude
Torralba et al,[31,32] 2010[a] Los Angeles, CA	PGY1-3 IM residents, n = 100	Rheumatologic emergencies, RA, SpA, OA, PM/DM, STR, CIA	Modified TBL: preclass preparation, in-class IRAT, GRAT, case application	ITE scores, cumulative attendance IRAT, GRAT, VOTS, classroom engagement survey	Knowledge, attitudes, reaction
Mok et al,[33] 2013 Hong Kong	MBBS IV, MBBS V; N = 124	Systemic lupus erythematosus	PBL, along with lectures, textbook, patient contact (mix)	Needs assessment Curriculum review	Attitude, reaction
Cannella et al,[34] 2015 Omaha, NE	MS2, n = 124	Gout, patient encounters, injections	Multiple: PBL, CBL, Augenblick cases, video game (gout), simulation laboratory (injections), patient encounters	Survey	Attitude, reaction
Law et al,[35] 2014[a] Atlanta, GA	MS3 (N not specified)	Critical thinking, cost consciousness	Decision-based learning in teams	Survey	Reaction
Guillen-Astete et al,[36] 2017 Madrid, Spain	MS2	Back pain	PBL	Review of medical registries: adherence to image test recommendations, treatment recommendations, need for further consultation	Behavior, reaction

(continued on next page)

Table 3
(continued)

Author/Year/Location	Learner Population	Topics	Interventions	Assessments	Outcome (Fitzpatrick Model[b])
Scott & Battafarano,[37] 2015 Houston, TX	IM residents, N-65	Arthrocentesis, various conditions	PBL/CBL, ARS, patient encounters, simulation	Before-after curriculum knowledge self-assessment, preference	Knowledge, reaction
Emery & Gardner,[38] 2010 Hayward & Emery,[39] 2017 Hayward et al,[40] 2016 Seattle, WA	MS2, varied blocks, 6 teaching sites	Includes RA, gout, JIA, SLE cases, pathology, imaging	Lectures with small group discussion of cases; 14 15-min stations	Multiple choice test, survey	Reaction, attitude, knowledge
El-Mediany et al,[41] 2019 Dartford, Kent, United Kingdom	Medical students, n = 55	(Topics not specified)	Preclass preparation, in-class activity	OSCE, satisfaction, and effectiveness survey	Knowledge, skills, reaction

Educational programs and training initiatives that use various teaching techniques but do not specify use of group-based activities were excluded from this table, and may be found elsewhere in this issue. Please refer to articles related to OSCEs (See Lisa Criscione-Schreiber's article, "Turning Objective Structured Clinical Examinations (OSCEs) into Reality," in this issue) and musculoskeletal medicine training (See Michael J. Battistone and colleagues' article, "Interprofessional Musculoskeletal Education: A Review of National Initiatives from the Department of Veterans Affairs," in this issue).

Abbreviations: ARS, audience response system; CBL, case-based learning; CIA, crystal-induced arthropathies; GRAT, group readiness assessment test; IM, internal medicine; IRAT, individual readiness assessment test; MBBS, medicinae baccalaureus chirurgiae; MS, medical student; OSCE, objective structured clinical examination; PBL, problem-based learning; PGY, postgraduate year; PM/DM, polymyositis/dermatomyositis; RA, rheumatoid arthritis; SpA, spondyloarthropathies ; STR, soft tissue rheumatisms; TBL, team-based learning.

^a This work was supported by an ACR/REF Clinician Scholar Educator Award. Note: Emery's original work 2010 was supported by this award, but the flipped classroom was applied thereafter.

^b Fitzpatrick levels of outcomes: patient health, change in patients' health; behavior, change in behavior (inclusion of skill in clinical practice); skills, change in skills (OSCE scores, observed assessment scores); knowledge, change in knowledge (written examination scores); attitudes, change in attitudes/perceptions (confidence self-ratings, comfort self-ratings); reaction, learner reaction (satisfaction with teaching method, satisfaction with instructor).

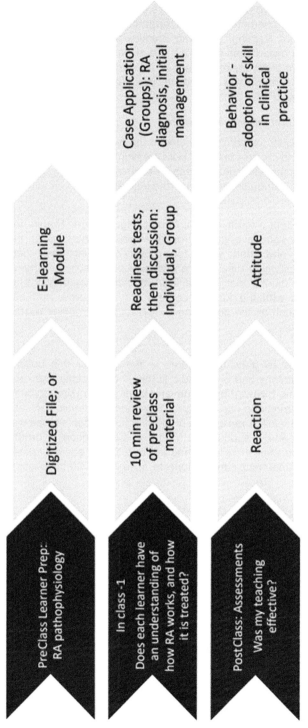

Fig. 3. Schema for modified TBL format for a noon core curriculum session on rheumatoid arthritis (RA) for internal medicine residents.

of portfolios has been explored for use in rheumatology fellowship training. Portfolios can be used not only to provide summative evidence of knowledge and procedural skills (nononcologic chemotherapy logs, arthrocentesis logs) but also to provide evidence of formative learning, including practice-based learning and improvement (practice reviews, case-based questions and research) and reflections.[65] With regard to the assessment of faculty effectiveness, an evaluation tool that identifies specific classroom-based approaches was developed that offers guidance to faculty on teaching strategies.[66]

Conundra: Incorporating Active Learning

The stakes are higher for learning situated in the real-world health care environment. Critical thinking and clinical reasoning skills are high-priority teaching goals. Therefore, when considering the educational cases presented, a didactic lecture may be insufficient without using strategies to engage the learner.

Case 1

Educators can adopt a modified TBL format (**Fig. 3**). After 15 minutes of deliberations, educators can have groups display their answers all at the same time using placards, and then ask each group regarding their decision-making process, thus facilitating discussions and also being able to obtain feedback as to the level of additional learning gained. Educators may survey the residents on their satisfaction with the format, content of the session, and use of specific learning points such as the screening for cytopenias and liver dysfunction before methotrexate use.

Case 2

A system change to prevent fractures is the goal for this collaborative effort between rheumatology and orthopedic surgery. A morbidity and mortality conference may be done, followed by the development of a working committee to review the medical literature, and use quality improvement strategies such as the Plan-Do-Study-Act (Practice). The development of a fracture liaison service was decided on as a means to prevent subsequent fractures. Comparison of practice habits for 1 year before and after the start of the fracture liaison service related to initiation of osteoporosis treatment can be done to assess the effectiveness of this active learning process.

ACKNOWLEDGMENTS

The authors acknowledge Beatrice Boateng, PhD, Department of Pediatrics, Arkansas Children's Hospital, University of Arkansas, Little Rock, AR; and Ron Ben-Ari, MD, former Program Director, University of Southern California (USC)–Los Angeles County Internal Medicine Residency Program, and Associate Dean for Continuing Medical Education, Keck School of Medicine, USC, Los Angeles, CA. Drs. Boateng and Ben-Ari contributed to Dr Torralba's project on Team Based learning. Funding for this project was provided by the Rheumatology Research Foundation Clinician Scholar Educator Award.

REFERENCES

1. Institute of Medicine. Crossing the quality chasm: a new health system for the 21st century. Washington, DC: The National Academies Press; 2001. Available at: https://doi.org/10.17226/10027.

2. Holmboe ES, Edgar L, Hamstra S. The milestones guidebook. Available at: https://www.acgme.org/Portals/0/MilestonesGuidebook.pdf. Accessed March 4, 2019.
3. Dharamsi S, Ho A, Spadafora SM, et al. The physician as health advocate: translating the quest for social responsibility into medical education and practice. Acad Med 2011;86:1108–13.
4. The Royal College of Physicians and Surgeons of Canada. CanMEDS: better standards, better physicians, better care. Available at: http://www.royalcollege.ca/rcsite/canmeds/canmeds-framework-e. Accessed March 4, 2019.
5. Adams NE. Bloom's taxonomy of cognitive learning objectives. J Med Libr Assoc 2015 Jul;103(3):152–3.
6. Anderson LW, Krathwohl DR, Airasian PW, et al. A taxonomy for learning, teaching and assessing: a revision of Bloom's. New York: Longman; 2001.
7. Miller GE. The assessment of clinical skills/competence/performance. Acad Med 1990;63:S63–7.
8. Kirkpatrick DL, Kirkpatrick JD. Evaluating training programs: the four levels. 3rd edition. San Francisco (CA): Berrett-Koehler; 2006.
9. Freeman S, Eddy SL, McDonough M, et al. Active learning increases student performance in science, engineering, and mathematics. Proc Natl Acad Sci U S A 2014;111(23):8410–5.
10. Taylor DCM, Hamdy H. Adult learning theories: implications for learning and teaching in medical education: AMEE Guide No. 83. Med Teach 2013;35(11): e1561–72.
11. Medina MS. Making students' thinking visible during active learning. Am J Pharm Educ 2017;81(3):41.
12. Fornari A, Poznanski A. How-to guide for active learning, vol. 39. Huntington, VA: Books; 2015. Available at: https://academicworks.medicine.hofstra.edu/books/39. Accessed March 8, 2019.
13. Merritt C, Munzer BW, Wolff M, et al. Not another bedside lecture: active learning techniques for clinical instruction. AEM Educ Train 2018;2(1):48.
14. Wiles AM. Figure analysis: a teaching technique to promote visual literacy and active Learning. Biochem Mol Biol Educ 2016;44:336–44.
15. Thambu N, Balakrishnan V. Forum theatre technique: enhancing learning in moral education classroom. Malays Online J Educ Manag 2014;2:53–69.
16. Melo Prado H, Hannois Falbo G, Rodrigues Falo A, et al. Active learning on the ward: outcomes from a comparative trial with traditional methods. Med Educ 2011;45:273–9.
17. Accreditation Council for Graduate Medical Education. ACGME program requirements for graduate medical education in rheumatology (internal medicine) 2017. Available at: https://www.acgme.org/Portals/0/PFAssets/ProgramRequirements/150_rheumatology_2017-07-01.pdf?ver=2017-04-27-153540-583. Accessed March 9, 2019.
18. Risko EF, Anderson N, Sarwal A, et al. Everyday attention: variation in mind wandering and memory in a lecture. Appl Cogn Psychol 2012;26:234–42.
19. Risko EF, Buchanan D, Medimorec S, et al. Everyday attention: mind wandering and computer use during lectures. Comput Educ 2013;68:275–83.
20. Ewers RM. Do boring speakers really talk for longer. Nature 2018;561(7724):464.
21. Novak JD. Meaningful learning: the essential factor for conceptual change in limited or inappropriate propositional hierarchies leading to empowerments of learners. Sci Educ 2002;86(4):548–71.

22. Vallori AB. Meaningful learning in practice. J Educ Hum Dev 2014;3(4):199–209. Available at: https://doi.org/10.15640/jehd.v3n4a18. Accessed March 8, 2019.
23. Chen WK, Wang P. A framework of active learning by concept mapping. US China Educ Rev 2012;11:946–52.
24. Michael J. Where's the evidence that active learning works? Adv Physiol Educ 2006;30:159–67.
25. Bowen JL. Educational strategies to promote clinical diagnostic reasoning. N Engl J Med 2006;355:2217–25.
26. Lubarsky S, Dory V, Audetat MC, et al. Using script theory to cultivate illness script formation and clinical reasoning in health professions education. Can Med Educ J 2015;6(2):e61–70.
27. Peña A. The Dreyfus model of clinical problem solving skills acquisition: a critical perspective. Med Educ Online 2010;15. https://doi.org/10.3402/meo.v15i0.4846.
28. Berrett D. How 'flipping' the classroom can improve the traditional lecture. The Chronicle of Higher Education. Available at: https://people.ok.ubc.ca/cstother/How_Flipping_the_Classroom_Can_Improve_the_Traditional_Lecture.pdf. Accessed March 8, 2019.
29. Cattaneo KH. Telling active learning pedagogies apart: from theory to practice. J New Approaches in Educational Research 2017;6(2):144–52. Available at: https://files.eric.ed.gov/fulltext/EJ1151062.pdf. Accessed March 8, 2019.
30. Scheers-Masters J, Blumenthal DR, Macrae J, et al. A Controlled pilot study on the use of active learning techniques during a rheumatology elective for medical residents. Abstract Number 1593. 2011 ACR/ARHP Annual Meeting. Arthritis Rheum 2011;63(10):S622. Available at: https://acrabstracts.org/wp-content/uploads/2018/06/2011_ACR_ARHP_Abstract_Supplement.pdf. Accessed March 8, 2019.
31. Torralba KD, Boateng BA, Ben-Ari R, et al. Team-based learning in rheumatology resident education: two-year results on receptiveness and attitudes of residents towards collaborative learning and teamwork. Abstract Number 46. ACR/ARHP 2010 Annual Meeting, Atlanta, GA. Arthritis Rheum 2010;62(10):S17. Available at: https://acrabstracts.org/wp-content/uploads/2018/06/2010_ACR_ARHP_Abstract_Supplement.pdf. Accessed March 8, 2019.
32. Torralba KD, Boateng BA, Ben-Ari R, et al. Abstract 3324: "effect of internal medicine resident participation in team-based learning on in-training exam scores in Rheumatology. Abstract Number 1432. ACR/ARHP 2010 Annual Meeting, Atlanta, GA. Arthritis Rheum 2010;62(10):S595. Available at: https://acrabstracts.org/wp-content/uploads/2018/06/2010_ACR_ARHP_Abstract_Supplement.pdf. Accessed March 8, 2019.
33. Mok MY, Lo Y, Lau CS. A needs assessment and review curriculum of content of teaching on systemic lupus erythematosus. Abstract Number 971. 2013 ACR/ARHP Annual Meeting. Available at: https://acrabstracts.org/abstract/a-needs-assessment-and-review-curriculum-of-content-of-teaching-on-systemic-lupus-erythematosus/. Accessed March 8, 2019.
34. Cannella AC, Moore GF, Mikuls TR, et al. Teaching rheumatology in undergraduate medical education: what are the students saying? [abstract]. Arthritis Rheumatol 2015;67(suppl 10). Available at: https://acrabstracts.org/abstract/teaching-rheumatology-in-undergraduate-medical-education-what-are-the-students-saying/. Accessed March 8, 2019.
35. Law K, Pittman JR, Miller C. Using Decision-Based Learning to highlight rheumatic disease for third-year medical students. Arthritis Rheumatol 2014;

66(1Suppl 20):S1259. Available at: https://acrabstracts.org/abstract/using-decision-based-learning-to-highlight-rheumatic-disease-for-third-year-medical-students/. Accessed March 8, 2019.

36. Guillen-Astete CA, Braña-Cardeñosa A, Zamorano-Serrano M, et al. BOP0066 The problem based learning applied to teaching rheumatological topics among non rheumatology residents. Ann Rheum Dis. Available at: https://doi.org/10.1136/annrheumdis-2017-eular.3984. Accessed March 8, 2019.

37. Scott J, Battafarano D. Assessment of a rheumatology curriculum utilizing multiple learning modalities [Abstract]. Arthritis Rheumatol 2015; 67(suppl 10). Available at: https://acrabstracts.org/abstract/assessment-of-a-rheumatology-curriculum-utilizing-multiple-learning-modalities/. Accessed March 8, 2019.

38. Emery H, Gardner G. "Rheumapalooza": An intensive rheumatology curriculum for second year medical students. Abstract 1433. ACR/ARHP 2010 Annual Meeting, Atlanta, GA. Arthritis Rheum 2010;62(10):S594. Available at: https://acrabstracts.org/wp-content/uploads/2018/06/2010_ACR_ARHP_Abstract_Supplement.pdf. Accessed March 8, 2019.

39. Hayward K, Emery HM. Rheumapalooza: a rheumatology curriculum in evolution [abstract]. Arthritis Rheumatol 2017;69(supp I4). Available at: https://acrabstracts.org/abstract/rheumatolooza-a-rheumatology-curriculum-in-evolution/. Accessed March 8, 2019.

40. Hayward K, Gardner G, Emery HM. Rheumatolooza update: applying a flipped classroom instructional model to an intensive rheumatology curriculum for second year medical students [abstract]. Arthritis Rheumatol 2016;68(suppl 10). Available at: https://acrabstracts.org/abstract/rheumapalooza-update-applying-a-flipped-classroom-instructional-model-to-an-intensive-rheumatology-curriculum-for-second-year-medical-students/. Accessed March 8, 2019.

41. El-Mediany Y, El-Gaafary M, El-Aroussy N, et al. Flipped learning: can rheumatology lead the shift in medical education? Curr Rheumatol Rev 2019;15(1): 67–73.

42. Wilson AS, Goodall JE, Ambrosini G, et al. Development of an interactive learning tool for teaching rheumatology – a simulated clinical case studies program. Rheumatology (Oxford) 2006;45(9):1158–61.

43. Battistone MJ, Barker AM, Grotzke MP, et al. Effectiveness of an interprofessional and multidisciplinary musculoskeletal training program. J Grad Med Educ 2016; 8(3):398–404.

44. Davis MH, Harden RM. AMEE medical education guide No 15. Problem based learning: a practical guide. Med Teach 1999;21:130–40.

45. Parmelee D, Michaelson LK, Cook S, et al. Team-based learning: a practical guide: AMEE Guide No. 65. Med Teach 2012;34(5):e275–87.

46. Yoong J, Lui NL. Educating future learners of rheumatology. PoSH 2013;22(1): 15–9. Available at: https://journals.sagepub.com/doi/pdf/10.1177/201010581302200104. Accessed March 8, 2019.

47. Sawatsky AP, Zickmund SL, Berlacher K, et al. Understanding resident learning preferences within an internal medicine noon conference lecture series: a qualitative study. J Grad Med Educ 2014;6:32–8.

48. Sawatsky AP, Zickmund SL, Berlacher K, et al. Understanding the challenges to facilitating active learning in the resident conferences: a qualitative study of internal medicine faculty and resident perspectives. Med Educ Online 2015;20: 27289. Available at: https://doi.org/10.3402/meo.v20.27289.

49. Bonwell CC, Eison JA. Active learning: creating excitement in the classroom. Washington DC: ERIC Digests; 1991. ED340272. Available at: https://files.eric.ed.gov/fulltext/ED340272.pdf. Accessed March 8, 2019.
50. Portnoy DB, Han PKJ, Ferrer RA, et al. Physicians' attitudes about communicating and managing scientific uncertainty differ by perceived ambiguity aversion of their patients. Health Expect 2011;16:362–72.
51. Adams S, Bilimoria K, Malhotra N, et al. Effort and trust: the underpinnings of active learning. Adv Physiol Educ 2017;41:332–7.
52. Deal CL, Hooker R, Harrington T, et al. The United States rheumatology workforce: supply and demand, 2005–2025. Arthritis Rheum 2007;56(3):722–9.
53. National Resident Matching Program. Match results statistics: medical specialties matching program – 2018. Appointment Year; 2019. Available at: https://mk0nrmpcikgb8jxyd19h.kinstacdn.com/wp-content/uploads/2018/11/Match-Results-Statics.pdf. Accessed March 8, 2019.
54. Goldenberg DL, Mason JH, De Horatius R, et al. Rheumatology education in United States medical schools. Arthritis Rheum 1981;24(12):1561–6.
55. Sheikh S, Smith M, Ning T, et al. Rheumatology decision 2011: factors influencing career decisions among rheumatology fellows. Abstract Number 1594. ACR/ARHP 2010 Annual Meeting, Atlanta, GA. Arthritis Rheum 2010;62(10):S622. Accessed March 8, 2019.
56. Miloslavsky EM, Criscione-Schreiber LG, Jonas BL, et al. Fellow as teacher curriculum: improving rheumatology fellows' teaching skills during inpatient consultation. Arthritis Care Res (Hoboken) 2016;68(6):877081. Available at. https://onlinelibrary.wiley.com/doi/epdf/10.1002/acr.22733. Accessed March 8, 2019.
57. Searle NS, Thibault GE, Greenberg SB. Faculty development for medical educators: current barriers and future directions. Acad Med 2011;86(4):405–6.
58. Archer J, McManus C, Woolf K, et al. Without proper research funding, how can medical education be evidence based? BMJ 2015;350:h3445.
59. Dolmans DHJM, Van Der Vleuten CPM. Research in medical education: practical impact on medical training and future challenges. GMS Z Med Ausbild 2010;27(2).
60. Collins C. Rheumatology pearls. Available at: http://www.rheumpearls.com/index.php. Accessed March 8, 2019.
61. American College of Rheumatology. Rheum4Science. Available at: https://www.rheumatology.org/learning-center/educational-activities/view/id/881. Accessed March 8, 2019.
62. Bauman A. Concept maps: active learning assessment tool in a strategic management capstone class. Coll Teach 2018;66(4):213–21.
63. Tomaswick L, Marcinkiewicz J. Active learning – concept maps. Kent State University Center for Teaching and Learning; 2018. Available at: https://www.kent.edu/sites/default/files/file/Teaching%20Tools%20In%20a%20Flash%20-%20Concept%20Maps.pdf. Accessed March 8, 2019.
64. MedEdPortal. Association of American Medical Colleges. The journal of Teaching and Learning Resources. https://www.mededportal.org. Accessed March 8, 2019.
65. Torralba KD, Boateng BA, Ben-Ari R, et al. Abstract 3367: "development of an ACMGE core competency-based electronic portfolio at the USC-LAC Rheumatology Fellowship Program". Abstract Number 3367. ACR/ARHP 2010 Annual Meeting, Atlanta, GA. Arthritis Rheum 2010;62(10):S595.

Available at: https://acrabstracts.org/wp-content/uploads/2018/06/2010_ACR_ ARHP_Abstract_Supplement.pdf. Accessed March 8, 2019.

66. Frankl S, Newman L, Burgin S, et al. The case-based collaborative learning peer observation worksheet and compendium: an evaluation tool for flipped classroom facilitators. MedEdPORTAL 2017;13:10583. Available at: https://doi.org/10. 15766/mep_2374-8265.10583. Accessed March 8, 2019.

Turning Objective Structured Clinical Examinations into Reality

Lisa Criscione-Schreiber, MD, MEd

KEYWORDS

- Observed structured clinical examination • OSCE • Clinical assessment • Simulation
- Communication • Education

KEY POINTS

- Objective structured clinical examinations evaluate learners "showing how" to perform complex clinical tasks including those infrequently observed and those core to rheumatology practice.
- Carrying out a rheumatology objective structured clinical examination requires multiple resources and must therefore provide worthwhile information if undertaken by training programs or institutions.
- Summative rheumatology objective structured clinical examinations as part of certification require extensive validity testing; rheumatology objective structured clinical examinations used in US fellowships thus far provide formative feedback to improve performance.
- Establishing validity and ensuring reliability is important in all objective structured clinical examinations and crucial if the rheumatology objective structured clinical examination is high stakes or summative.
- Although trainees find rheumatology objective structured clinical examinations stressful, steps can be taken to maximize their potential as positive formative learning experiences.

WHAT IS AN OBJECTIVE STRUCTURED CLINICAL EXAMINATION?

Objective structured clinical examinations (OSCEs) are performance assessments, first described in the 1970s[1] and now in widespread use as assessment tools in medical education. A concise OSCE description follows:

> An assessment tool based on the principles of objectivity and standardization, in which the candidates move through a series of time-limited stations in a circuit for

Disclosure Statement: The author has received funding from Rheumatology Research Foundation Clinician Scholar Educator Career Development Award in the year 2011-2014.
Division of Rheumatology and Immunology, Program for Women in Internal Medicine, Department of Medicine, Duke University School of Medicine, Box 3490 DUMC, 40 Duke Medicine Circle, Durham, NC 27710, USA
E-mail address: lisa.criscione@duke.edu

Rheum Dis Clin N Am 46 (2020) 21–35
https://doi.org/10.1016/j.rdc.2019.09.010
0889-857X/20/© 2019 Elsevier Inc. All rights reserved.

the purposes of assessment of professional performance in a simulated environment. At each station candidates are assessed and marked against standardized scoring rubrics by trained assessors.[2]

An OSCE is one tool available to medical educators to assess learners' ability to perform complex tasks that involve knowledge, behaviors, skills, and attitudes. On Miller's pyramid[3] of assessment, OSCEs reside at the "shows how (in simulated environments)" level, the penultimate measurement, just under the complexity assessed by observing "does" (**Fig. 1**). Learners' clinical skills are evaluated in OSCEs during multiple short ($\leq$15 minutes), focused, simulated practice experiences in which the learner participates as the primary provider. OSCEs are designed with the ideal that the only variable is the learner who rotates from station to station. Thus, in each OSCE station, the learner faces the same clinical scenario and rating format, with individual stations in a circuit using the same standardized patient and the same rater. The structured clinical examination part of the name indicates that the purpose of an OSCE is as an assessment in which the participant is rated or graded. These assessments can be formative, with a learner receiving feedback for the purpose of improving future performance, or summative, meaning the OSCE results are used to make determinations of success such as promotion, graduation, or board certification (eg, the US Medical Licensing Examination Step 2 Clinical Skills Assessment).[4] OSCEs consist of multiple stations such that through observing performance in different scenarios a full picture of a learner's skills emerges.

Obviously, there are myriad ways individual learners' clinical competency can and should be assessed, including observation of actual patient interactions. The

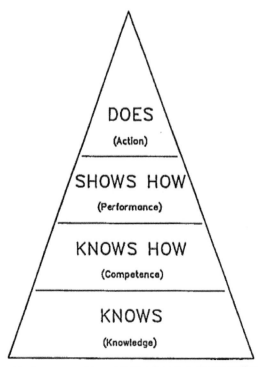

Fig. 1. Miller's pyramid of assessment in medical education. (*From* Miller GE. The assessment of clinical skills/competence/performance. Acad Med 1990;65(9 Suppl):S63; with permission.)

use of assessment through standardized cases, however, allows for scoring against a rubric and/or the opportunity to compare performance between learners. Such scoring rubrics often include checklists of behaviors that should be performed to receive credit for completion. Although checklists are helpful, it should be noted that global rating systems also have good reliability.[5] Because expert clinicians use shortcuts, including efficient questioning to quickly narrow the differential diagnosis and arrive at the correct management plan, experts may not ask every question on a scoring checklist and may score lower than novices on such rating systems. Owing to such potential pitfalls, most OSCEs are scored using a combination of station-specific checklists and global ratings. As a test of clinical performance, scoring based on preset criteria (criterion referenced) rather than scoring through comparison with other participants' performance (norm referenced) is preferred.[6] Both validity and scoring reliability in OSCEs can be improved through scoring rubrics and training both raters and standardized patients. When executed appropriately and well, OSCEs represent an informative component of a global assessment schema that ensures documented clinical competence of medical trainees. For the purposes of this article, we refer to a rheumatology OSCE as a ROSCE.

WHEN SHOULD A RHEUMATOLOGY OBJECTIVE STRUCTURED CLINICAL EXAMINATION BE USED?
To Assess "Shows How"

Referring to Miller's pyramid,[3] in medical education one should choose the type of assessment that matches the level of performance requiring assessment. Medical knowledge is efficiently assessed using multiple choice tests. Essay questions or oral examinations can reveal how well a learner "knows how" to incorporate medical knowledge into more complex situations. Simulations such as an OSCE reveal how well complex situational understanding translates into observable behaviors. Direct observation of clinical care is the highest level, assessing "does." Although direct observations in patient care are highly important, some clinical scenarios are foundational to each medical subspecialty, or are unusual but crucially important for a clinically competent practitioner. For example, in rheumatology, fellows in training are rarely observed responding to telephone inquiries from patients or other providers, or may benefit from feedback after observing key skills such as counseling patients with new rheumatologic diagnoses or when changes in high risk biologic medications are indicated. A multistation ROSCE is a good way to assess multiple learners' performance in such clinical scenarios.

WHEN THE ASSESSMENT'S VALUE MERITS THE REQUIRED LABOR, PERSONNEL, SPACE, AND TIME

Even when performed routinely, every OSCE is labor intensive. Planning includes deciding on station objectives, writing clinical scenarios, creating rating forms, and recruiting and training standardized patients and examiners, as well as arranging logistics.[5] Each OSCE involves many individuals, determined by the number of stations and learners. Each station requires a standardized patient and a rater; recorded stations can be rated later, but that still requires a significant time investment by the evaluator. The experience of an OSCE is fairly intense: standardized patients, learners, and proctors all get tired after a couple hours; a station may require a change in patient if consecutive circuits are run (or when managing the schedules of busy medical professionals).

Where to administer an OSCE can be a challenge. Although there are facilities at most medical schools for circuit-based simulations, even technology enhanced with a central observation area and time keeper, running the actual OSCE requires humans to be available in case anything goes awry as well as making sure all supplies stay in place, learners go to the correct stations, and all the technology is working. Simulation space may be unavailable or prohibitively expensive for use by rheumatology training programs, in which case medical educators must either use actual clinic space (prohibiting simultaneous patient care) or create a simulated clinic space elsewhere. An OSCE requires multiple examination rooms large enough to accommodate a learner, 1 or more standardized patients, and an observer (in-person observer, 1-way mirror, or camera).

In addition to preparation time, administering an OSCE can take several hours. Complex clinical scenarios require up to 30 minutes per station with additional time (1–5 minutes) for learners to transition between stations. For example, an 8-station ROSCE for 24 fellows, run in 3 circuits with 15 minutes per station plus transfer will take at least 2 hours to complete if 3 circuits are run simultaneously. More learners need more circuits; whether in shifts or simultaneously, requiring more planning, personnel, and time or space.

An assessment that merits the described investments has to result in gaining information that cannot be effectively assessed in other (easier) ways. We know OSCEs are best used to assess communication skills, professionalism skills, or clinical reasoning skills in specific clinical scenarios.[7] A ROSCE can be an efficient way to assess multiple learners in scenarios they all encounter, such as counseling patients about risks of disease-modifying antirheumatic drugs or dealing with a hostile patient. As medical educators, we have all faced the challenge of trying to get our faculty members to directly observe trainees in clinical practice. Thus, it is highly possible that any individual fellow will not be observed performing core patient counseling tasks during the course of their 2- to 3-year training period. In a ROSCE, we can observe each trainee's performance in multiple standard clinical scenarios during one period of time. In addition to counseling on standard clinical scenarios, OSCEs can be used to assess performance and interpretation of core rheumatology skills such as the musculoskeletal examination,[8] or to identify opportunities for improvement in counseling or professionalism skills in sometimes challenging patient situations.[9]

WHAT DATA SUPPORT THE USE OF OBJECTIVE STRUCTURED CLINICAL EXAMINATION IN RHEUMATOLOGY EDUCATION?
Musculoskeletal Examination

Several published reports about OSCEs in rheumatology have assessed musculoskeletal examination skills. One publication described 2 well-validated stations to assess medical student performance of the hand and knee examination[10] that correlated with performance in a multistation physical examination OSCE. Another described a single station that assessed physical examination of the shoulder and knee[11] and another evaluated examination of the shoulder, knee and hands in a UK postgraduate rheumatology nursing program.[12] This publication is of special interest in view of the recently published curriculum for training Nurse Practitioners and Physician Assistants for rheumatology practice[13] suggesting that OSCEs could be used to assess competence when training advanced practice providers. Recently, Battistone and colleagues[8] published their validation process for an OSCE assessing the specific musculoskeletal examination skills needed to evaluate shoulder and knee pain, specifically to identify rotator cuff and meniscal pathology. This OSCE assessing practical diagnostic skills was one component of a unified curriculum to teach examination skills to primary care providers in the US Department of Veterans Affairs and monitor how this educational program impacts the appropriateness and cost of care for these conditions.

Musculoskeletal Ultrasound Examination

A ROSCE has been developed and conducted for several years to assess participants' ability to perform and interpret musculoskeletal ultrasound examiantions.[14] This 9-station OSCE began as a summative assessment following a year-long correspondence course on musculoskeletal ultrasound examinations. To assess validity, the authors compared OSCE performance results to scores on a 76-item multiple choice question test. Each OSCE station was graded live by a proctor and remotely by 2 additional raters using a checklist. The authors compared upper quartile and lower quartile performers on the multiple choice question test to those same individuals' OSCE performance using Pearson's correlation test and found that the groups correlated. Additionally, composite OSCE scores discriminated the bottom quartile fellows from course faculty when assessing normal wrists and ankles but not on stations with abnormal joints. Of interest, the inter-rater reliability was acceptable (0.7) between the remote assessors, but live proctors and remote assessors had a lower inter-rater reliability of only 0.3 with proctor scores routinely higher than those of the remote raters. The authors postulated this difference in scoring was either due to the benefit of observing the real-time acquisition of images or to the challenge of simultaneously observing and rating, and concluded that remote blinded grading increased reliability. This finding is potentially relevant to other OSCEs; it may be difficult for an individual to both proctor and score a station simultaneously, so there may be benefit to remote scoring, especially if the OSCE is summative or high stakes. Additionally, the interpersonal interaction, although minimal, in a live OSCE may make it more challenging for a rater to score the test taker critically.

RHEUMATOLOGY FELLOW PERFORMANCE: SUMMATIVE

An early described experience trialed a ROSCE as a summative component of clinical competency assessment among individuals in 1 region of the UK completing their rheumatology training.[15] This 13-station ROSCE included interactions with real trained patients (interviewing, counseling, and examination) as well as skill stations such as radiograph and synovial fluid interpretation, scored live by faculty raters. Informal feedback was given to the 12 participants after all ROSCE stations were completed. In summary, the authors found the ROSCE gave useful information to the committee that decided on awarding trainees with a Certificate of Completion of Specialist Training in Rheumatology, when considered along with several other performance evaluations.

More recently, the Mexican Accreditation Council for Rheumatology described their validation and use of a ROSCE as a component of their certification process along with a 300-item multiple choice question examination.[16] Because this OSCE is for summative certification purposes, this group compared both a criterion-referenced pass mark and setting the passing standard based on the borderline performance method. Candidates' performance seemed to be better using criterion-referenced passing than the borderline performance method, although ultimately both scoring methods correlated well with the multiple choice question score.[17] In this OSCE, the authors found generally high communication skills scores; patients scored communication higher than the physician examiners, and communication scores correlated with the overall scoring on each station. Of interest, the group reported that the average communication skill score weakly correlated with multiple choice question score.[18]

RHEUMATOLOGY FELLOW PERFORMANCE: FORMATIVE

There is support for the use of OSCEs as formative assessments and learning opportunities, especially because establishing acceptable reliability for a high-stakes evaluation is complex and resource intensive.[19] Most US rheumatology training programs have few faculty members and enroll 1 or 2 fellows annually, making the conduct of a ROSCE challenging, so regional rheumatology training programs collaborate to conduct ROSCEs.

Berman and colleagues[20] described the first 5 years of experience with an annual formative ROSCE designed to primarily assess communication and professionalism skills among New York City fellowship program trainees. Their project goals included being able to document meaningful fellow improvement over the 2-year training program and comparison of ROSCE scores with the training directors' pre-ROSCE assessments of their own fellows. Learners received a global rating on each station as well as individual items by both a standardized patient and a live faculty proctor. Verbal feedback from both faculty and standardized patients was given at the completion of each ROSCE station. Fellows demonstrated improvement between years with roughly similar scores across individual fellows (did not reach statistical significance) and program directors rated their own fellows higher before the OSCE than the ROSCE raters (program directors did not proctor their own fellows) did. Program directors did consistently distinguish higher and lower performing fellows. After the aforementioned experience, the New York group developed more psychosocially or medically complex scenarios and reported on identification of verbal and nonverbal skills that best correlated with high professionalism scores. Physician raters scored professionalism lower than patient actors did, and the groups seemed to value different elements of professionalism. Qualitative analysis revealed that physician raters frequently commented on body language and word choice, how a plan was articulated, and shared decision making. Higher use of medical jargon negatively correlated with professionalism scores for both patient actor and faculty raters; perception of empathy by both patient actors and faculty correlated ($r = 0.7$) well with overall professionalism scores and inversely with use of jargon.[9] This New York City ROSCE is a continued annual collaboration between programs to provide formative feedback to fellows on communication and professionalism skills.

Similarly, the Carolinas Fellows Collaborative (CFC) has conducted an annual ROSCE since 2006 as a low-stakes formative evaluation with stations covering all 6 Accreditation Council of Graduate Medical Education competencies and immediate feedback after each station. This ROSCE has also been used to assess important clinical skills that may be undertaught in rheumatology fellowships, such as rehabilitation medicine and management of infusion reactions. Aggregate fellow performance on such ROSCE stations can identify programmatic areas in need of development for trainee education; such ROSCE stations have been followed by targeted educational interventions such as live didactic sessions on infusion reactions[21] and an online spaced education program on exercise recommendations for patients with arthritis.[22]

For the first several years of the CFC ROSCE, trainees were not given information about expected content. Although this allowed us to assess what fellows knew about the management of certain clinical scenarios without preparation, we found that poor performance on hard stations did not lead the same fellow to improve the following year (unpublished data), suggesting that poor performance did not drive increased study. In addition, on post-OSCE surveys some fellows felt their performance was hampered by unclear expectations and inadequate preparation. Recognizing that fellows prepare for uncomfortable or unusual patient scenarios before actual patient visits, since 2015 we have provided fellows with descriptions of each station 1 week before the ROSCE to allow preparation. As has been reported,[23] this simple change seems to have decreased stress associated with the ROSCE and increased the perception among fellows that it is a useful part of their rheumatology training (unpublished data). However, some fellows do not seem to take the opportunity to prepare, which begs the question of what about the OSCE stimulates learning? For many, the act of testing with direct observation seems to drive a desire to do their best and thus prepare for the OSCE. Others seem to prefer researching areas of poor performance after the exercise, some seem unmotivated by this exercise and prefer learning driven by other motivators.

Although OSCEs are not in widespread use among adult rheumatology fellowship programs, they are even more unusual among pediatric rheumatology programs, which are smaller and more geographically diverse than adult programs. Within the past decade some highly dedicated medical educators in pediatric rheumatology organized 2 national pediatric ROSCEs (PROSCEs) at the American College of Rheumatology Annual Scientific Meetings. The 7 scenarios focused on patient counseling in scenarios such as describing risks of steroids, counseling about specific diagnoses, musculoskeletal examination, and joint injection techniques.[24] Per their checklist results, they identified some specific items that were omitted by many fellows and altered their scoring system between 2009 and 2011 administrations. Postadministration evaluations reflected widespread acceptance of the PROSCE as a formative educational assessment by the pediatric rheumatology fellow participants with ongoing plans for a PROSCE to be offered national meetings (Megan Curran, MD, personal communication, 2019).

ARE THERE POTENTIAL HAZARDS TO USING AN OBJECTIVE STRUCTURED CLINICAL OBJECTIVE STRUCTURED CLINICAL EXAMINATION FOR PERFORMANCE ASSESSMENT?

The main risk of any OSCE is in how a learner accepts and reacts to this performance assessment. Although performance in the setting of an examination should result in a best performance,[7] learners report anxiety leading up to and during OSCEs.[25,26] Actual or perceived poor performance resulting in negative feedback or constructive feedback given poorly could hurt a learner's confidence or self-esteem. As an example, after a CFC ROSCE we surveyed fellows regarding their perceived compared with typical performance in similar real situations. No fellows thought their performance on the ROSCE was much better than their usual performance; when surveyed immediately after the ROSCE and at 4 months after, fellows generally felt their performance on the ROSCE was either typical (41% immediate, 40% remote) or worse than their typical performance (59% immediately, 53% remotely) (Criscione-Schreiber L, 2014, unpublished data). Only 1 fellow responded that their ROSCE performance was somewhat better than their usual performance, and only on the survey 4 months later. For fellows who reported their performance was different from their usual performance, we further asked, "To what do you attribute this difference [in performance]?" Among responses received, elements of fellows' comments could be placed into 6 categories, including unclear expectations, nervousness, artificial situation, inadequate preparation, time pressure, and being watched or videotaped. These findings are similar to other published concerns from learners.[25,26] As noted elsewhere in this article, in response to these findings we now send a description of the ROSCE stations ahead of time to allow fellows to prepare a best performance. Although the OSCE is a simulation, it does present real possible scenarios, so even if fellows are adapting their learning to fit the assessment method, the skills practiced should be transferrable to future direct patient care.

Other hazards of OSCEs relate more to the definition of knowledge being assessed, given that rating forms assume that the faculty know and define what is correct and incorrect in each scenario, thus running the risk of preserving the status quo. When observing rheumatology fellows who have already been physicians for more than 3 years, faculty members should be open to learning from fellows' unique approaches and broadening the set of possible correct answers or approaches. Noting that OSCEs can identify systemic patterns of practice within an institution, an OSCE could identify practices that mis-shape learning.

Although the adult learners in rheumatology fellowship programs appreciate the ROSCEs educational value, they do not generally enjoy the experience. Immediately after the ROSCE, close to one-quarter of participants reported they enjoyed it not at all, with 65% enjoying it either only slightly or somewhat, and only 12% enjoying it very much. The numbers improved somewhat when queried 4 months later, but 14% still reported they enjoyed the ROSCE not at all, 64% reported they enjoyed it only slightly or somewhat, and 21% reported they enjoyed it very much (unpublished data). We have not formally surveyed faculty about their responses to the ROSCE, but other published reports support our observation that proctoring an OSCE is tiring.[15] Overall, the results of an OSCE must be considered among many assessments appropriately chosen to give a comprehensive picture of performance.

HOW VALUABLE IS AN OBJECTIVE STRUCTURED CLINICAL EXAMINATION AS A FORMATIVE ASSESSMENT?

To answer this question, we queried fellows about the CFC ROSCEs perceived educational value, predicting fellows would (1) agree it was a useful educational activity and (2) find the ROSCE more educationally valuable when viewing it in retrospect. We tallied responses to immediate and 4-month (remote) post-ROSCE surveys. Both immediately and remotely, fellows generally agreed the ROSCE helped them to gain a better understanding of both their specific strengths and weaknesses in medical knowledge, patient care, and interpersonal and communication skills. As predicted, the percentage of participants who rated the ROSCE as either very helpful or somewhat helpful in identifying strengths or weaknesses was higher when assessed remotely than immediately; the only ratings of not at all helpful were given on the survey taken immediately after the ROSCE. When surveyed months later, no fellows rated the ROSCE as not at all helpful, and fewer respondents rated the ROSCE as only somewhat helpful in identifying strengths and weaknesses. Additionally, all participants at least somewhat agreed with the statement that the ROSCE stations were sufficiently representative of rheumatology practice. All participants at least somewhat agreed they had received useful feedback from both standardized patients and faculty proctors, with similar percentages strongly agreeing, somewhat agreeing, and agreeing immediately and 4 months after the ROSCE. Finally, we asked fellows, "Overall, how would you rate the educational effectiveness of the ROSCE for you?" No fellows reported the ROSCE to be not at all effective. Values were similar at both time points, with 83% immediately and 87% months later agreeing that the ROSCE was either somewhat or very educationally effective (**Fig. 2**).

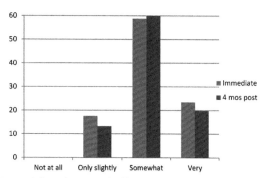

Fig. 2. Fellows' ratings of the educational effectiveness of the rheumatology objective structured clinical examination (ROSCE) in response to the question "Overall, how would you rate the educational effectiveness of the ROSCE for you?" The y-axis shows the percentage of fellows selecting each response at the immediate (*blue*) and remote, 4 months after ROSCE (*red*) time points.

During the PROSCEs that were offered nationally in 2009 and 2011, pediatric rheumatology fellow participants were also queried about their perception of the PROSCEs value as an educational activity. The authors reported that 85.7% of participants answered that they would change some aspect of their clinical behavior based on feedback received. In addition, after both administrations the average rating was about 75 of 100 on a visual analog scale regarding the overall value of the PROSCE.[24]

Simulations give opportunity to make mistakes and get feedback without impacting patient care. Proctoring an OSCE helps educators to internalize the value of direct performance observation with insight into how trainees' competence is evaluated. Giving structured feedback in an OSCE helps to develop these skills for use after the OSCE. At a programmatic level, a ROSCE can highlight areas in which all trainees need additional education and practice. Additionally, during a formative OSCE trainees see their teachers' dedication to their education in action. Medical educators are dedicated to the success of their trainees. Conducting a ROSCE is one way to invest in each learner's training with structured feedback to improve performance. Ultimately, this feedback should lead to improved capability of our trainees to communicate effectively and provide highly professional clinical care to patients with rheumatic diseases.

HOW DOES ONE DESIGN AN OBJECTIVE STRUCTURED CLINICAL EXAMINATION WITH VALIDITY?

Validity means that an assessment tool measures what it is designed to measure. Reliability, or the reproducibility of the test results, is an important goal when creating evaluations that enhances the validity of an assessment. Validity also refers to how test results are used, ensuring their use is commensurate with the importance and design of the assessment.[2]

OSCE validity starts with design. For appropriate development, the AMEE Guide no. 81 describes the history and theoretic background of OSCEs (part I)[2] and the nuts and bolts of how to design one (part II),[5] as well measuring an OSCEs quality in AMEE Guide no. 49.[27] First, one must decide which concepts will be assessed (eg, professionalism, clinical reasoning, or other skills and behaviors). OSCEs are not the best tool to assess medical knowledge, which can be measured in a number of other ways, including multiple choice question testing. Create an OSCE blueprint with competencies and concepts as column headers and planned stations as rows. Ideally, there should be redundancy in concepts assessed across stations to give more opportunities for participants to be assessed in each.

Both validity and reliability increase with a greater number of stations and using standardized scoring rubrics, trained examiners, and standardized patients.[2] Whether using actual patients or patient actors, the standardized patients must be trained to behave similarly through multiple iterations of the same station.[2] Medical schools generally have available patient actors accustomed to playing such roles, although the cost may be prohibitive.

For scoring, one may use checklists (yes/no vs numerical ratings), rating scales, global ratings, or a combination thereof (**Table 1**). Recall that, for experts (rheumatology trainees should be expert clinicians by fellowship), global ratings show better reliability than checklists.[5] Behavioral checklists are best developed by panels of experts, as has been done in rheumatology for several potential OSCE stations,[28] and can document what has been done, but not necessarily how well. Rating scales of behaviors tend to be more subjective than checklists, so scoring rubrics with behavioral anchors can improve reliability.[7] Overall, however, global rating scales tend to show the greatest reliability when observing clinical care scenarios.[5]

Station descriptions and scoring rubrics should be reviewed by several medical educators for clarity and to ensure the station has been designed to effectively evoke the desired competencies and behaviors for assessment. Stations should be piloted to ensure objectives can be met in the allotted time, the interaction makes sense and scoring forms are clear. Piloting a station gives an opportunity to discuss types of behaviors that merit different scoring levels (behavioral anchors) for reliability.

High-stakes OSCEs must include a passing standard and proof of validity. Because individual checklist items are codependent and contribute to overall station performance, each station should receive an aggregated score. That said, checklist items across a single domain, such as communication, can be compared across stations to give an average domain score for the entire OSCE.[7] As described elsewhere in this article, criterion-referenced passing standards are preferable to norm-referenced. Within criterion-referenced scoring, the Angoff and Ebel methods can be used, although were both developed for scoring multiple-choice examinations where there is a known correct answer. Thus, they may be useful for OSCEs assessing procedural performance such as musculoskeletal ultrasound examiantions,[14] but less so for clinical interactions. Other methods for setting passing standards include the borderline group and contrasting groups methods,[5,7] detailed discussion of which are beyond the scope of this review.

In summative OSCEs, both internal consistency and inter-rater reliability should be determined. Internal consistency, or Cronbach's α, refers to the test's ability to discriminate the higher performing from lower performing examinees and should be at least 0.7[27] for high-stakes examinations. For inter-rater reliability (the kappa statistic), values of greater than 0.60 represent substantial agreement and those between 0.41 and 0.60 moderate agreement. Acceptance of either of these levels of agreement should be determined by the stakes of the assessment, certainly greater tha 0.60 for any high-stakes examination.[29]

SHOULD I USE A RHEUMATOLOGY OBJECTIVE STRUCTURED CLINICAL EXAMINATION IN MY FELLOWSHIP TRAINING PROGRAM?

An OSCE represents an opportunity for feedback on clinical skills and for medical educators to demonstrate dedication to improving patient care outcomes by ensuring consistent and effective practices among trainees. Fellows value the feedback given.

Table 1
Items on a faculty proctor scoring sheet for a patient counseling station of the CFC ROSCE focused on the clinical scenario of preconception counseling for a patient with systemic lupus erythematosus

	1 Fellow Demonstrated This Skill, Behavior, or Attitude Not at All	2 Fellow Demonstrated This Skill, Behavior, or Attitude Occasionally	3 Fellow Demonstrated This Skill, Behavior, or Attitude Most of the Time	4 Fellow Demonstrated This Skill, Behavior, or Attitude Always
Listening				
Fellow allowed patient to freely ask questions				
Fellow allowed patient to speak uninterrupted				
Fellow's questions and statements reflected listening				
Verbal communication				
Introduced self in respectful/friendly manner				
Used language patient could understand				
Answered patient's questions				
Interaction progressed in a logical order				
Fellow provided information at a level of understanding for the patient				
Fellow summarized and/or indicated the next steps				
Body language				
Appearance/manner appropriate				
Maintained eye contact				

Systems-Based Practice	1 Yes	2 No		
Fellow acknowledged the importance of communication with the patient's current providers				
Fellow assured patient of communication with current providers				
Global Ratings	1 Poor	2 Fair	3 Good	4 Excellent
Interpersonal communication skills				
Systems-based practice skills				
Entire counseling station				
Comments:				

Although a large multistation ROSCE may seem daunting for small or geographically isolated programs, OSCE-style simulations with 1 to 2 stations at a time should be achievable by even small programs. Such mini-ROSCEs could feasibly be conducted a few times a year by a couple of dedicated faculty members. Regardless of setting, it is important that rheumatology trainees be directly observed performing clinical duties to attest to their competency and continually develop their skills through coaching.

In the United States, there are ongoing discussions about subspecialty certification and maintenance thereof. Currently, certification in rheumatology by the American Board of Internal Medicine requires the training program director to affirm that each graduate is competent to practice rheumatology independently and without supervision based on Accreditation Council of Graduate Medical Education milestones assessments performed every 6 months during training. This sign-off makes graduates eligible to take the American Board of Internal Medicine Rheumatology Certification Examination, a rigorously designed and validated multiple choice question test. Including an OSCE among routine training assessments provides 1 more piece of evidence to support an affirmation of clinical competency. Although OSCEs are currently part of initial physician certification in the United States (United States Medical Licensing Examination Step 2), Internal Medicine certification by the Royal College of Physicians and Surgeons of Canada and are included in rheumatology certification in Mexico, much work would need to be done to validate an OSCE for national use in the United States. Currently in the United States, even for procedures such as endoscopy, echocardiography, and rheumatology musculoskeletal ultrasound examination, certification requires documentation of completed procedures in addition to a multiple choice question examination but not directly observed procedure performance by the certifying body. If a certification ROSCE were to be developed, it would require significant investment by the certifying board, including evidence that the results of such an examination would be able to identify incompetent rheumatologists, who should not practice owing to low scores correlating with poor patient care outcomes.

SUMMARY

In summary, a ROSCE can be used to evaluate trainees performing multiple clinical and other activities to observe behaviors and interactions that are considered essential to the practice of rheumatology. Conducting a ROSCE requires a group of dedicated medical educators and significant time investment and logistical support. Although an OSCE is stressful for the trainee, our adult learners generally appreciate the value of observed simulated interactions for obtaining formative feedback to improve performance. Although a summative ROSCE may be appropriate in certain settings to assess clinical competency for licensure, a formative ROSCE is useful for assessing both individual trainees as well as the efficacy of the training program as a whole. When creating an OSCE, careful design is important to maximize validity and reliability, especially if the OSCE becomes summative or high stakes. Participating in an OSCE as a medical educator is an opportunity to participate in the training of learners to provide optimal patient care. As we create and administer OSCEs to our learners, we are contributing to the development of a workforce to most effectively care for individuals with rheumatic diseases.

DISCLOSURE

The author has no relevant disclosures.

REFERENCES

1. Harden RM, Stevenson M, Downie WW, et al. Assessment of clinical competence using objective structured examination. Br Med J 1975;1(5955):447–51.
2. Khan KZ, Ramachandran S, Gaunt K, et al. The Objective Structured Clinical Examination (OSCE): AMEE guide no. 81. Part I: an historical and theoretical perspective. Med Teach 2013;35(9):e1437–46.
3. Miller GE. The assessment of clinical skills/competence/performance. Acad Med 1990;65(9 Suppl):S63–7.
4. Gormley G. Summative OSCEs in undergraduate medical education. Ulster Med J 2011;80(3):127–32.
5. Khan KZ, Gaunt K, Ramachandran S, et al. The Objective Structured Clinical Examination (OSCE): AMEE guide no. 81. Part II: organisation & administration. Med Teach 2013;35(9):e1447–63.
6. Takayesu JK, Kulstad C, Wallenstein J, et al. Assessing patient care: summary of the breakout group on assessment of observable learner performance. Acad Emerg Med 2012;19(12):1379–89.
7. Yudkowsky R. In: Downing SM, Yudkowsky R, editors. Assessment in health professions education. New York: Routledge; 2009. p. 217–45.
8. Battistone MJ, Barker AM, Beck JP, et al. Validity evidence for two objective structured clinical examination stations to evaluate core skills of the shoulder and knee assessment. BMC Med Educ 2017;17(1):13.
9. Berman JR, Aizer J, Bass AR, et al. Fellow use of medical jargon correlates inversely with patient and observer perceptions of professionalism: results of a rheumatology OSCE (ROSCE) using challenging patient scenarios. Clin Rheumatol 2016;35(8):2093–9.
10. Raj N, Badcock LJ, Brown GA, et al. Design and validation of 2 objective structured clinical examination stations to assess core undergraduate examination skills of the hand and knee. J Rheumatol 2007;34(2):421–4.
11. Vivekananda-Schmidt P, Lewis M, Coady D, et al. Exploring the use of videotaped objective structured clinical examination in the assessment of joint examination skills of medical students. Arthritis Rheum 2007;57(5):869–76.
12. Ryan S, Stevenson K, Hassell AB. Assessment of clinical nurse specialists in rheumatology using an OSCE. Musculoskeletal Care 2007;5(3):119–29.
13. Smith BJ, Bolster MB, Slusher B, et al. Core curriculum to facilitate the expansion of a rheumatology practice to include nurse practitioners and physician assistants. Arthritis Care Res (Hoboken) 2018;70(5):672–8.
14. Kissin EY, Grayson PC, Cannella AC, et al. Musculoskeletal ultrasound objective structured clinical examination: an assessment of the test. Arthritis Care Res (Hoboken) 2014;66(1):2–6.
15. Hassell AB, West Midlands Rheumatology Services and Training Committee. Assessment of specialist registrars in rheumatology: experience of an objective structured clinical examination (OSCE). Rheumatology (Oxford) 2002;41(11):1323–8.
16. Pascual Ramos V, Medrano Ramirez G, Solis Vallejo E, et al. Performance of an objective structured clinical examination in a national certification process of trainees in rheumatology. Reumatol Clin 2015;11(4):215–20.
17. Pascual-Ramos V, Guilaisne Bernard-Medina A, Flores-Alvarado DE, et al. The method used to set the pass mark in an objective structured clinical examination defines the performance of candidates for certification as rheumatologists. Reumatol Clin 2018;14(3):137–41.

18. Pascual-Ramos V, Flores-Alvarado DE, Portela-Hernandez M, et al. Communication skills in candidates for accreditation in rheumatology are correlated with candidate's performance in the objective structured clinical examination. Reumatol Clin 2019;15(2):97–101.

19. Losh D. The value of real-time clinician feedback during OSCEs. Med Teach 2013;35(12):1055.

20. Berman JR, Lazaro D, Fields T, et al. The New York City Rheumatology Objective Structured Clinical Examination: five-year data demonstrates its validity, usefulness as a unique rating tool, objectivity, and sensitivity to change. Arthritis Rheum 2009;61(12):1686–93.

21. Weiner JJ, Eudy AM, Criscione-Schreiber LG. How well do rheumatology fellows manage acute infusion reactions? A pilot curricular intervention. Arthritis Care Res (Hoboken) 2018;70(6):931–7.

22. Patel A, O'Rourke K. A primer on exercise: an interactive, online educational module incorporating spaced education to supplement the ACR core curriculum outline for rheumatology fellowship programs. Arthritis Rheumatol 2017;69(suppl 10) [abstract].

23. Barry M, Noonan M, Bradshaw C, et al. An exploration of student midwives' experiences of the Objective Structured Clinical Examination assessment process. Nurse Educ Today 2012;32(6):690–4.

24. Curran ML, Martin EE, Thomas EC, et al. The pediatric rheumatology objective structured clinical examination: progressing from a homegrown effort toward a reliable and valid national formative assessment. Pediatr Rheumatol Online J 2019;17(1):5.

25. Nasir AA, Yusuf AS, Abdur-Rahman LO, et al. Medical students' perception of objective structured clinical examination: a feedback for process improvement. J Surg Educ 2014;71(5):701–6.

26. Pierre RB, Wierenga A, Barton M, et al. Student evaluation of an OSCE in paediatrics at the University of the West Indies, Jamaica. BMC Med Educ 2004;4:22.

27. Pell G, Fuller R, Homer M, et al. How to measure the quality of the OSCE: a review of metrics - AMEE guide no. 49. Med Teach 2010;32(10):802–11.

28. Criscione-Schreiber LG, Sloane RJ, Hawley J, et al. Expert panel consensus on assessment checklists for a rheumatology objective structured clinical examination. Arthritis Care Res (Hoboken) 2015;67(7):898–904.

29. Axelson RD, Kreiter CD. Reliability. In: Downing SM, Yudkowsky R, editors. Assessment in health professions education. New York: Routledge; 2009. p. 57–74.

Online Resources for Enhancing Clinical Knowledge and Skills

Megan L. Curran, MD[a],*, Kristen Hayward, MD, MS[b],
Jay Mehta, MD, MSEd[c]

KEYWORDS

- E-learning • Online • Education • Rheumatology • Musculoskeletal • Pediatric

KEY POINTS

- Online educational resources offer practicing rheumatologists flexible, easy access to learning opportunities for ongoing professional development.
- Online resources can connect learning communities and provide virtual feedback to distance learners.
- Limitations of online learning include weak evidence for skill acquisition and behavior change, and the need for maintenance to ensure currency and user interface functioning.

INTRODUCTION

"E-learning" is an overarching term used since the 1980s[1] referring not only to instruction occurring via digital media,[1–3] but also to a flexible, engaging and learner-centered pedagogical approach.[4] During the rise of the Internet in the 1990s, medical educators were encouraged to embrace technology to develop innovative instructional methods.[5] Advantages of e-learning methods include that they provide opportunities for distance learning, take advantage of economies of scale, allow for consistent messages, allow for flexible scheduling, provide individualized learning, use novel instructional methods, furnish assessment means, and document records of usage and assessment.[3]

Over the past 3 decades, medical education e-learning resources have exponentially expanded to include a large variety of instructional formats via the Internet and

[a] Section of Rheumatology, Children's Hospital of Colorado, University of Colorado School of Medicine, 13123 East 16th Street, Box 311, Aurora, CO 80045, USA; [b] Division of Rheumatology, Seattle Children's Hospital, University of Washington, School of Medicine, 4800 Sand Point Way Northeast, M/S MA.7.110, Seattle, WA 98105, USA; [c] Perelman School of Medicine at the University of Pennsylvania, Children's Hospital of Philadelphia, 3501 Civic Center Boulevard, CTRB 10109, Philadelphia, PA 19104, USA
* Corresponding author.
E-mail address: megan.curran@childrenscolorado.org

Rheum Dis Clin N Am 46 (2020) 37–60
https://doi.org/10.1016/j.rdc.2019.09.011
0889-857X/20/© 2019 Elsevier Inc. All rights reserved.

mobile devices. E-learning can be offered in a strictly digital format or via blended learning, when combined with in-person teaching. E-learning encompasses electronic articles, test question banks, tutorial modules, virtual patients, instructional videos, and massive online open courses. Each of these methods has been used to deliver rheumatology and musculoskeletal-focused content, which can supplement other educational methods like interactive small groups (see Best Evidence in Medical Education Guide No. 18, a systematic review about teaching musculoskeletal clinical skills).[6] Lim and Bolster[7] recently noted that optimizing medical education for practitioners is vital to maintain a competent workforce.

RESOURCE DEVELOPMENT AND ASSESSMENT

Guidelines for developing e-learning technology[8] and incorporating learning, teaching, and assessment methods[4] have been published by the Association of Medical Educators in Europe. When developing e-learning materials and choosing an instructional method, it is helpful to carefully consider the intended audience, including the stage and type of learner. A formal needs assessment of anticipated users is an important and often overlooked first step in resource development.[9] For rheumatology-specific content, learners range from preclinical students through practicing, board-certified providers and include not only physicians but also allied health professionals. Types of instructional resources range from those used by solitary learners to online courses that can engage groups of learners and in which direct instructor feedback and student discussion take place. It is imperative to incorporate a mechanism to evaluate whether the resource is achieving its intended purpose. Resources can be evaluated on 2 levels: assessment of learner knowledge, often measured by Miller's pyramid model,[10] and evaluation of the instructional program itself, often using the framework of Kirkpatrick and Kirkpatrick.[11] Both are outlined in **Table 1**.

For pragmatic reasons, it can be difficult to evaluate the true impact of educational resources on clinical skills in practice or population health. To facilitate ongoing resource evaluation and improvement, a quality improvement framework may be used to measure process-associated outcomes such as how instructional resources are used. The Standards for Quality Improvement Reporting Excellence (SQUIRE) guidelines, extension for education projects, outlines the steps to undertake when developing and publishing projects about systematic efforts to improve health professions education.[12] Another educational intervention evaluation method is qualitative analysis of data from participant feedback.

ONLINE RHEUMATOLOGY RESOURCES

There are many examples of e-learning resources in rheumatology, some supported by peer-reviewed publications demonstrating impact on learners' knowledge and skill acquisition. Resources are targeted at a variety of worldwide learners including trainees and practicing providers in medicine and allied health fields, all of whom have different learning goals.

Importantly, many resources seek to provide education on rheumatology and musculoskeletal medicine for the wider health professions workforce, not just for rheumatologists. Given the shortage of US specialist providers in both adult and pediatric rheumatology,[13] rheumatologists must help support primary care providers to recognize rheumatic and musculoskeletal diseases, conduct initial evaluation of patients, and make appropriate referrals. Technology and e-learning allow connection with the international medical workforce to a degree that is historically unprecedented. An organization supporting this effort is the Global Alliance for Musculoskeletal Health

Table 1					
Conceptual frameworks for learning outcomes and educational program evaluation					
	Miller,[10] 1990			Kirkpatrick & Kirkpatrick,[11] 2006	
	Learning Outcomes Assessment Model			Program Evaluation Model	
Level	Descriptor	Outcome	Descriptor	Outcome	
1	Knows	Learner's factual knowledge	Reaction	Learner's reaction to an instructional resource	
2	Knows how	Learner's application of facts	Learning	Learner's factual knowledge	
3	Shows	Learner's demonstration of knowledge/skills	Behavior	Learner's behavior in clinical practice	
4	Does	Learner's performance of skills	Results	Impact on patient populations	

of the Bone and Joint Decade,[14] which notes a worldwide shortage of musculoskeletal providers and advocates for accessible educational methods for frontline providers.

Tables 2–7 feature selected e-learning resources grouped by location and format. Resources were identified through a PubMed search using combinations of the terms "online, "e-learning," "mobile applications," "rheumatology," "pediatric," and "education," as well as a review of existing medical education resource catalogs: the Association of American Medical College's MedEdPORTAL[15] and OuchMyLeg!,[16] a Web site to curate and share pediatric rheumatology content. OuchMyLeg! provides a virtual hub to foster collaboration and sharing of teaching materials for educators within this underserved subspecialty.[17]

Professional Society Resources

Several professional societies have played a notable role in development of electronic resources dedicated to ongoing professional development in rheumatology; examples are noted in **Table 2**.

European League Against Rheumatism

European League Against Rheumatism (EULAR) has a strong history of assessing the rheumatology community's educational needs. A survey of various stakeholders in postgraduate rheumatology education throughout Europe highlighted barriers to accessing continuing education. Specifically, they identified lack of time and resources to attend educational programs, as well as variability in language of learners as significant barriers. Online courses were cited as a potential viable platform to address the need for flexible, easy access to ongoing professional development.[18]

In response to the needs of its membership, EULAR developed the EULAR Online Course on Rheumatic Diseases.[19] Managed by a scientific course committee, this completely Internet-based course provides roughly 210 hours of educational training targeted toward practicing rheumatologists. This course was successfully piloted with a 10-module subcourse and 70 trial learners and has been expanded to accommodate 50 modules designed to be completed over a 2-year course. Feedback has been very positive; most respondents to a survey about EULAR resources indicated that resources adequately met their educational needs.[20] Successful completion after passing a final examination is recognized by certificate. Another example of a European online course in rheumatology is a master's degree curriculum for postgraduate education offered entirely online through the University of South Wales.[21]

Table 2
Rheumatology educational resources provided by professional societies

Resource Name	Link	Author or Sponsoring Society	Target Audience	Description	Assessment Method Available
ACR Online Courses[22]	https://www.rheumatology.org/Learning-Center/Educational-Activities	American College of Rheumatology (ACR)	Students, residents, fellows, attending and allied health professionals; must be ACR member to access	Fundamentals of rheumatology, advanced rheumatology course and shorter intermediate and advanced level e-Bytes modules, including slide sets, word documents with "pearls" and podcasts	Posttests; continuing medical education credit available
Rheum2Learn[54]	https://www.rheumatology.org/Learning-Center/Educational-Activities/Rheum2Learn	American College of Rheumatology	Internal medicine program directors and residents; rheumatology health professionals	Web-based rheumatology self-study modules mapped to the 6 core American College of Graduate Medical Education competencies	Posttest
Rheum4Science[55]	https://www.rheumatology.org/Learning-Center/Educational-Activities/View/ID/881	American College of Rheumatology	Students, residents, fellows, attendings	Case-based modules to teach clinical research methodology and fundamental immunology necessary for rheumatology practice	Posttests
High Impact Rheumatology[56]	https://www.rheumatology.org/Learning-Center/Educational-Activities/High-Impact-Rheumatology	American College of Rheumatology	Primary care providers	PowerPoint-based curriculum with goals of increasing knowledge and management skills regarding treatment for arthritis and musculoskeletal diseases	None

Continuing Assessment Review Evaluation (CARE)	https://www.rheumatology.org/Learning-Center/Educational-Activities	American College of Rheumatology	Rheumatology trainees and physicians	Multiple-choice questions written by rheumatologist educators with detailed answer explanations to assess and improve knowledge	Yes
EULAR School of Rheumatology[19]	https://esor.eular.org/theme/lc_eular/layout/home/course.php?id=35	European League Against Rheumatism	Physicians and health professionals	50-module online course designed to be completed in 2 years with registration fee	Yes including final examination
Versus Arthritis[57]	https://www.versusarthritis.org/about-arthritis/healthcare-professionals/	Arthritis Care and Arthritis Research UK; Royal College of General Practitioners	Students, health professionals, especially general practitioners	Information about arthritis and musculoskeletal pain: videos, free 5-h e-learning module "Core skills in MSK Care," patient education resources	Resources to demonstrate how learning has impacted patient care; quizzes
PREP Rheumatology[27]	https://shop.aap.org/2019-prep-rheumatology/	American Academy of Pediatrics	Rheumatology trainees and health professionals	Fee-based multiple-choice board examination-style questions	Yes

Table 3
Rheumatology educational resources created by Rheumatology Research Foundation Clinician Scholar Educator awardees

Resource Name	Link	Author or Sponsoring Institution	Resource Type	Target Audience	Description
OuchMyLeg![16]	https://ouchmyleg.northwestern.edu/	Megan Curran; Northwestern University	Web site	Pediatric rheumatologists; educators	Pediatric rheumatology and musculoskeletal teaching materials sharing network Web site; chief resident community within site can allow residency training programs to access materials but not currently active
A Competency Based Musculoskeletal Ultrasound Curriculum[26]	http://www.ussonar.org/	Eugene Kissin, et al	Musculoskeletal ultrasound curriculum	Rheumatology fellows and attendings	Teaching materials, quizzes and ultrasound image submission for review and 20-h course on how to standardize and improve scanning technique
A Modular Curriculum in Pediatric Rheumatology for Residents, Pediatricians and Adult Specialists[58]	https://pediatrics.mc.vanderbilt.edu/interior.php?mid=10605	Amy Woodward; Vanderbilt University School of Medicine Department of Pediatrics	Case study modules	Pediatric trainees and pediatricians	Case studies about joint hypermobility, knee pain, juvenile dermatomyositis, and pediatric psoriatic arthritis

Table 4
Rheumatology education Web sites

Resource Name	Link	Author or Sponsoring Institution	Target Audience	Description
Pediatric-education.org[59]	https://pediatriceducation.org/casesbyspecialty/	Donna and Michael D'Alessandro	Pediatric trainees	Curated collection of pediatric cases, some rheumatology, searchable by disease, specialty and symptom; text-based cases with patient presentation, discussion and learning points
RheumaKnowledgy[60]	http://www.rheumaknowledgy.com/	John J. Cush, Arthur Kavanaugh, C. Michael Stein	Medical and other health professions trainees or practitioners	Free online rheumatology textbook with 3 main sections: diagnosis, diseases, drugs and treatment
Pediatric Musculoskeletal Matters International[61]	http://www.pmmonline.org	Newcastle University and Northumbria University	Nurses, student nurses, doctors and clinicians	Information about clinical assessment, investigations, pain by site; includes key references, guidelines, algorithms, links to useful Web sites, patient and general practitioner information sheets, videos; includes content for global/international audiences
Univadis: everyday essentials for the modern clinician[62]	https://www.univadis.com/home/education?kw=keyword_rheumatology	Aptus Health, a subsidiary of Merck & Co., Inc.	Physicians and health professionals	Free medical education and news community whose Web site includes rheumatology information in various content formats including courses, expert presentations, quizzes and patient cases

(continued on next page)

Table 4
(continued)

Resource Name	Link	Author or Sponsoring Institution	Target Audience	Description
Enthesitis and enthesopathy[63]	http://enthesis.info/	Dennis McGonagle, Michael Benjamin	Health professionals	Information about enthesis anatomy and pathophysiology
Practice Improvement using Virtual Online Training[64]	https://www.the-pivot-project.org/	American College of Rheumatology, The Lupus Initiative	Students, physicians, and other health care professionals	Case-based game that aims to teach about the clinical reasoning processes and pitfalls in the diagnosis of lupus
JIA Calculator[65]	http://www.jra-research.org/JIAcalc/	Edward Behrens, The Children's Hospital of Philadelphia	Health professionals	Calculator to categorize patients with juvenile idiopathic arthritis into the correct International League of Associations for Rheumatology classification subtype
Introduction to Pediatric Musculoskeletal Clinical Skills - pGALS[66]	https://cpd.ncl.ac.uk/courses/course-details/2	Pediatric Musculoskeletal Matters, Newcastle University	Health professionals; particularly targeted at medical students	Free 30-min course providing knowledge to support musculoskeletal assessment of children and adolescents in primary and secondary care
Pediatric Musculoskeletal Medicine in Primary Care[67]	https://cpd.ncl.ac.uk/courses/course-details/5	Helen Foster, Sharmila Jandial, et al.; Newcastle University	Primary care clinicians	Free 40-min course with practical tips to support assessment of pediatric musculoskeletal presentations and direct further management of children and young people; Certificate of Completion

Resource	URL	Source/Author	Audience	Description
E-medicine pediatric rheumatology articles[68]	https://emedicine.medscape.com/pediatrics_general	Medscape	Health care professionals	Text-based short review articles written by pediatric rheumatologists, covering background, pathophysiology, etiology, epidemiology, prognosis, patient education, presentation, differential diagnosis, workup, treatment, guidelines and medications
Emedicine adult rheumatology articles[69]	https://emedicine.medscape.com/rheumatology	Medscape	Health care professionals	Text-based short review articles written by pediatric rheumatologists
Rheumatology Mind Map[70]	http://rheumatologymindmap.com/	Alex Papou	Health care professionals	Facts about rheumatic conditions organized using a mind map model
Rheumtutor[71]	http://www.rheumtutor.com/	Raj Carmona	Learners at all stages of medical training	Text-based information about diseases, investigations, assessment tools, medications, musculoskeletal examination, injection techniques and clinical images

Table 5
Rheumatology educational modules

Resource Name	Link	Authors	Target Audience	Description	Assessment Method Available; Outcomes and Impacts
Pediatric Rheumatology Curriculum for the Pediatrics Resident: A Case-Based Approach to Learning[72]	https://www.mededportal.org/publication/10767/	Miriah Gillispie, Eyal Muscal, Jennifer Rama, et al.	Pediatric and med-ped residents	Four 30-min case discussions, observed musculoskeletal examination session; designed to teach core skills (workup, physical examination, laboratory interpretation, and referral process) in pediatric rheumatology; published 2018	Likert scale participant self-report of comfort with workup laboratory interpretation, physical examination, and referral to rheumatology; before and after rotation (Kirkpatrick level 1); showed increase in resident comfort levels
Clinical Reasoning Workshop: Cervical Spine and Shoulder Disorders[73]	https://www.mededportal.org/publication/10560/	Alex Moroz	Physical medicine and rehabilitation residents	Interactive game-based workshop to improve clinical reasoning skills for patients presenting with shoulder and neck complaints; consists of small-group preparation followed by a case-based workshop; published 2017	Pretests and posttests on cases; reaction to session (Kirkpatrick 1 and 2; nonvalidated assessment tool); showed short-term improvement in knowledge; positive response
Development and Evaluation of a Web-Based Dermatology Teaching Tool for Preclinical Medical Students[74]	https://www.mededportal.org/publication/10619/	Moira Scaperotti, Nelson Gil, Ian Downs, et al.	Preclinical medical students	Case-based series of animated modules on dermatology topics, including cases on psoriasis and lupus, module posttest and survey; published 2017	29-question multiple-choice examination (Kirkpatrick 2); showed differential improvement in modular content for intervention arm

Resource	URL	Authors	Audience	Description	Assessment/Evaluation
PedsCases - A Learning Module for Evaluation of a Pediatric Limp for Medical Students[75]	https://www.mededportal.org/publication/7910/	Peter Gill, Peter MacPherson, Claire LeBlanc, et al.	Medical students in clinical training years	Podcast overview of the evaluation of the limping child and a case example with questions/answers; published 2010	No information on assessment of tool
PedsCases: A Learning Module for an Approach to Juvenile Idiopathic Arthritis for Medical Students[76]	https://www.mededportal.org/publication/10383/	Brieanne Rogers, Janet Ellsworth	Medical students in clinical training years	Podcast, reference chart, self-assessment tool, case examples covering basics of juvenile idiopathic arthritis; published 2010	No detailed information on specific assessment of tool
Examination of the Shoulder[77]	https://www.mededportal.org/publication/9551/	Henry Averns, Lindsay Davidson	Preclinical medical students	Module covering clinical assessment of shoulder pain, including anatomy, history, physical examination, pattern recognition, case study and a self-assessment quiz; published 2013	No assessment or evaluation data
Sam Rodilla, Knee Pain[78]	https://www.mededportal.org/publication/9078/	Ralitsa Akins, Kanchan Pema	Medical students	Standardized patent script, facilitator guide, OSCE checklist for patient with knee pain; published 2012	Case was assessed for interrater reliability: high at 80%
Low Back Pain Ambulatory Medicine Cases[79]	https://www.mededportal.org/publication/9565/	Arielle Berger, Parag Sheth, Sara Bradley	Clinical medical students, internal medicine and family medicine residents	Instructors guide for 1-h workshop; 3 back pain cases for students and faculty; published 2013	No assessment data; well received by students and facilitators
Structured Oral Examinations in Internal Medicine - Case H[80]	https://www.mededportal.org/publication/1120/	Hani Almoallim, Ali Alkatheeri, Alaa Monjed, et al.	Medical students	Case scenario about woman with lupus, laboratory data, images, OSCE checklist; published 2009	No assessment or evaluation data

(continued on next page)

Table 5
(continued)

Resource Name	Link	Authors	Target Audience	Description	Assessment Method Available; Outcomes and Impacts
Basic Skills in Musculoskeletal Examination: Hands-on Training Workshop[81]	https://www.mededportal.org/publication/9398/	Hani Almoallim, Doaa Kalantan, Mohammad Shabrawishi, et al.	Medical students, residents, attending physicians	Instructors guide for 3-h workshop to teach musculoskeletal examination skills, approach to early arthritis; student booklets with guide to regional examinations, case presentation slides; published 2013	No assessment or evaluation data
Joint Effusion Workshop[82]	https://www.mededportal.org/publication/10368/	Beth Rubinstein, Faizah Siddique	Medical students	Instructor's guide to case-based workshop on approach to joint effusions, workshop slides, synovial fluid chart; published 2016	Positive feedback from learners
Internal Medicine Clerkship Team-Based Learning Series: Joint Pain Module[83]	https://www.mededportal.org/publication/9147/	Steven Bishop, Jeffrey Kushinka, Stephanie Call	Medical students	90-min team-based learning module about approach to joint pain, with instructors guide, individual readiness assessment test, group readiness assessment; published 2012	No assessment or evaluation data

Internal Medicine Clerkship Team-Based Learning Series: Back Pain Module[84]	https://www.mededportal.org/publication/9153/	Steven Bishop, Jeffrey Kushinka, Stephanie Call	Medical students	90-min team-based learning module about approach to back pain with instructor's guide and group application cases; published 2012	No assessment or evaluation data
Hands-On Lightly Embalmed Cadaver Lab for Teaching Knee Aspiration/Injection[85]	https://www.mededportal.org/publication/9187/	Sarah Keim Janssen, Stephane P. VanderMeulen, Darwin Brown	Medical trainees	Training session on knee joint aspiration/injection with instructor guide, laboratory guide, slide presentation about technique; published 2012	No assessment or evaluation data
Pediatric Rheumatology Case-Based e-Learning Modules[86]	https://lpchrheum.moodlecloud.com/	Rosemary Peterson	Medical students and residents	Interactive computer-assisted case-based modules focused on core pediatric rheumatologic conditions	Self-study questions; prospective interventional study showed increased resident learner and fellow teacher satisfaction compared with traditional didactic slide format

Table 6
Selected rheumatology educational videos

Resource Name	Link	Author or Sponsoring Institution	Target Audience	Description
Musculoskeletal Gait Arms Legs Spine (GALS) examination video[87]	https://www.youtube.com/watch?v=b8eSqR9Pu24	Macleod's Clinical Examination	Health professionals	10-min video demonstrating GALS examination
GALS examination (Gait, Arms, Legs, Spine) - OSCE Guide[88]	https://www.youtube.com/watch?v=pClOlpzo-Jc	Lewis Potter, Geeky Medics	Health professionals	5-min video demonstrating GALS examination
Enthesitis examination video[89]	http://www.youtube.com/watch?v=xtOLGIm1hhU	David Sherry	Health care trainees and professionals	Video about entheseal anatomy and examination techniques

American College of Rheumatology/Rheumatology Research Foundation

Within the US rheumatology community, the American College of Rheumatology (ACR)/Rheumatology Research Foundation (RRF) has been a robust supporter of development of online rheumatology educational content. Resources developed or sponsored by the ACR are available on the ACR's Learning Center Web site[22] and are listed in **Table 2**. The ACR's educational efforts have been bolstered by a competitive RRF Clinician Scholar Educator (CSE) grant program.[23] The CSE award offers salary support for educational resource development and implementation, as well as financial support for project development and ongoing professional development in education. Awardees often undertake coursework within certificate and master's degree programs. Many CSE projects have developed electronic-based educational offerings.[24] **Table 3** shows selected publicly available CSE projects and resources.

As an example of a very successful CSE project, Kissin and colleagues[25] developed and implemented a blended approach to teaching rheumatologists basic musculoskeletal ultrasound, described elsewhere in this issue of *Rheumatic Disease Clinics*. The Ultrasound School of North American Rheumatologists course[26] that Dr. Kissin's project was applied toward, provides learners with a virtual online classroom space. The online portions of the course are supplemented by in-person experiences and an observed structured clinical examination for assessment of learner competency. Over the past 10 years, the course has produced more than 400 graduates, including adult and pediatric rheumatology fellows and faculty.

American Academy of Pediatrics

A professional society well-known for supporting provider education, the American Academy of Pediatrics (AAP) recently launched PREP Rheumatology,[27] a curriculum for board preparation for pediatric rheumatology fellows and continuing education for board-certified pediatric rheumatologists. The curriculum consists of a series of multiple-choice case-based questions with detailed answer explanations and

Table 7
Rheumatology education mobile applications

Resource Name	Link or Type	Author or Sponsoring Institution	Target Audience	Description
RheumPearls[90]	www.rheumpearls.com; https://twitter.com/RheumPearls	Christopher Collins	Medical students, residents and fellows	Web site lists more than 300 pearls of wisdom about rheumatology, all 140 characters or less. Twitter feed @RheumPearls
Essential Imaging in Rheumatology Clinical Case Challenge[91]	Mobile phone application	John M. O'Neill, Kim Legault	Health care trainees and professionals	Information from *Essential Imaging in Rheumatology* textbook[93] (Springer 2015) including diagnostic images, extended cases, short cases
Essential Imaging in Rheumatology Uncovering the Hand Radiograph[92]	Mobile phone application	John M. O'Neill, Stephany Pritchett	Health care trainees and professionals	Information from *Essential Imaging in Rheumatology* textbook[93] about radiographic basics, imaging anatomy, key imaging features, approach to interpretation, approach to clinical diagnosis
iAnkylosingSpondylitis[94]	Mobile phone application	Anatomate-Apps, humanmedia.net	Health care trainees and professionals	Short videos about ankylosing spondylitis, diagnosis, nonpharmacological management including diet and exercise and pharmacologic management
Rheumatology Advanced Vital Education[95]	Mobile phone application	Philip Mease, et al; DKBmed LLC; Nicholson NY, LLC; sponsors: Novartis, Bristol-Myers Squibb	Health care trainees and professionals; section for patients	Information about ankylosing spondylitis, psoriatic arthritis and rheumatoid arthritis, including classification criteria, calculators for disease activity scales

(continued on next page)

Table 7
(continued)

Resource Name	Link or Type	Author or Sponsoring Institution	Target Audience	Description
RheumaIQ[96]	Mobile phone application	Paulo Gobert	Health care trainees and professionals	Application providing rheumatology decision support that has calculators for disease classification criteria and disease activity indices
Essential Imaging in Rheumatology Unraveling Spondyloarthropathy[97]	Mobile phone application	John M. O'Neill, Christopher Russell	Health care trainees and professionals	Information from *Essential Imaging in Rheumatology* textbook[93] about ankylosing spondylitis, anatomy and imaging, diagnosis, alternate pathologies and case studies
@Point of Care Rheumatologic Diseases[98]	Mobile phone application	@Point of Care	Health care professionals	Text-based information about ankylosing spondylitis, juvenile idiopathic arthritis, psoriatic arthritis and rheumatoid arthritis written by rheumatologists with quiz questions and continuing medical education credit available
@RheumJC[99]	rheumjc.com; Twitter feed #RheumJC; https://twitter.com/RheumJC	Christopher Collins, Paul Sufka, Suleman Bhana, et al	Health care professionals	Virtual rheumatology journal clubs offered over Twitter
CORE: Clinical Orthopedic Examination[100]	Mobile phone application: http://clinicallyrelevant.com/core-clinical-orthopedic-exam/	Clinically Relevant Technologies	Health care trainees and professionals	Database of more than 400 clinical tests with descriptions on how to perform them, video demonstrations, diagnostic properties and links to supporting medical references

suggestions for further reading. Questions can be viewed on the AAP Web site or delivered to a mobile device.

Academic Educator Resources

In addition to electronic resources supported by larger organizations, academic educators have created e-learning rheumatology educational materials within Web sites (see **Table 4**) and online modules (see **Table 5**). In certain cases, findings related to implementation and assessment of the impact of these resources have been published.

Pediatric gait arms legs and spine

A site deserving particular recognition is Pediatric Musculoskeletal Matters (PMM),[28] whose chief editor is Dr Helen Foster. PMM is an evidence-based, online learning tool and information resource to raise awareness among general practitioners about pediatric musculoskeletal diseases, facilitate early diagnosis, and improve clinical outcomes.[28] Dr Foster and colleagues[29] created and validated the pediatric gait arms legs and spine (pGALS) examination, a quick series of maneuvers and questions to assess the pediatric musculoskeletal system designed for primary care providers to determine when to do further workup or refer to rheumatology or orthopedics. A series of videos and a mobile application were developed to teach the pGALS.[30]

Case studies for medical students

As another e-learning resource, rheumatologists at the University of Birmingham in the United Kingdom developed a series of 30 interactive online case studies involving patients with rheumatologic conditions. An initial study of undergraduate medical students using the cases indicated positive attitudes toward the educational materials. Students felt the cases were realistic, presented in an intuitive manner, and useful for their learning (Kirkpatrick level 1). To assess learning, students wrote a report based on one of the clinical cases regarding the information or actions relevant to the case and how they were used in the diagnosis or treatment. The reports were reviewed by rheumatologists and graded, with most learners earning a score of 70% or greater, demonstrating acquisition of knowledge from the intervention (Miller and Kirkpatrick levels 2). Unfortunately, these cases are not currently publicly available.

Rheumatology-dermatology education

An example of online rheumatologic disease education for dermatologists was recently published by Haemel and colleagues,[31] in which 3 case-based PowerPoint modules (cutaneous lupus and dermatomyositis, morphea and systemic sclerosis, and vasculitis) focus on clinical presentation, histology, pathophysiology, complication screening, therapy, medication monitoring, and outcome measures. Users' knowledge was significantly improved between pretesting and posttesting (Miller level 1), and learners felt the curriculum to be engaging, useable (Kirkpatrick level 1), and effective (Kirkpatrick level 2). Because patient photos are used in the modules, there are privacy concerns. Therefore the educational modules are only available through the members-only American Academy of Dermatology Web site.

Private Sector Resources

Private sector companies also contribute rheumatology-relevant e-learning resources. UpToDate[32] is an evidence-based, physician-authored clinical decision support aid, and is likely the most widely used private sector resource. DynaMed[33] is another clinical information resource designed to be used at the point of care. UpToDate and DynaMed are fee-based and require either institutional or individual subscription. In contrast, Medscape[34] and StatPearls[35] are publicly available, free resources authored by and aimed for physicians, containing relevant clinical information. StatPearls articles are indexed by PubMed, contain quiz questions to test learning, and offer continuing medical education credits for participation.

Social Media Platforms

Social media platforms can be harnessed to provide online resources for rheumatology learning.[7] The ability to share videos on Web sites such as YouTube[36] has created a shared repository of rheumatology educational material for visual and auditory learners, including musculoskeletal examination instruction. Some examples are outlined in **Table 6**. A publication by Fischer and colleagues[37] reviewed YouTube knee arthrocentesis videos and found most had good procedure technique but had a low-average score for educational value.

Other social media technology for e-learning includes mobile applications and Twitter accounts (see **Table 7**). Mobile applications are searchable in the Apple App Store[38] or Android Google Play[39] sites and include educational topics, such as musculoskeletal anatomy, rheumatic diseases, and classification criteria. Many, but not all, are free of charge. Twitter is an online messaging service in which members post short messages called tweets.[40] An introduction to Twitter for rheumatologists in slide show format is available online.[41] Various rheumatology educators and organizations manage Twitter accounts as a way to connect personally with learners. Examples include an account that publishes educational pearls about rheumatology[42] and another that sponsors virtual journal clubs.[43]

Challenges in E-Learning

Despite the appeal and desirability of e-learning tools and resources, there are important limitations. Most significantly, e-learning is not a substitute for hands-on clinical learning.[6] Questions remain as to when and where e-learning is appropriate to the task at hand, and what multimedia and high-fidelity resources add to learning. Another limitation is that electronic resources may not be distributed effectively or made publicly available.

In 2010, Wong and colleagues[44] undertook a qualitative systematic review of 249 papers to identify theory-driven criteria to guide the development and evaluation of Internet-based medical courses, with the objective of defining what e-learning resources work for whom and in what circumstance. Using Davis' Technology Acceptance Model[45] and Laurillard's model of interactive dialogue,[46] they found that learners were more likely to accept a course if it offered a perceived advantage over non-Internet alternatives, was easy to use technically, and compatible with their values and norms. When learners were able to use e-learning resources to communicate with an instructor, fellow students, or virtual tutorials and gain formative feedback, this interactivity led to effective learning. They identified 5 questions for learners to ask of an Internet-based course:[44]

1. *How useful will the e-learning technology be?* Will it increase your access to learning, provide consistent/high-quality content, be convenient, save you money or time? Are self-assessment methods available?
2. *How easy is the technology to use?*
3. *How well does this learning format fit in with what I am used to and expect?*

4. *How will high-quality human-human interaction be achieved?* Will there be structured virtual seminars, email, bulletin boards, real-time chat, supplementary media?
5. *How will feedback be achieved?* Are there questions with automated feedback or simulations?

Drawbacks of many videos and mobile applications reviewed herein include the fact that materials may not be peer-reviewed and that author attribution can be unclear. Additional disadvantages include inadequate technology, user distraction, and the potential for breakdown in barriers between personal and professional or educational use, which can present professionalism challenges.[47] In particular, use of an electronic platform does not ensure learner engagement. Some designs do not incorporate principles of effective learning, and in other cases, the technology itself may take a front role and obscure rather than enhance the content being delivered.[3]

For many online resources, there is a notable lack of data on assessment of learning outcomes[48,49]; this problem is common in medical education and not necessarily unique to e-resources.[50,51] The distance learning and relative anonymity of use of the electronic format may make it more difficult to collect ongoing substantive feedback from users without specific mechanisms in place to assess tool utilization and impact. Most of the rheumatology e-learning resources reviewed in this article do not have published outcomes about the effectiveness of the interventions, either at the learner or patient levels. When available, studies mostly show learner satisfaction with the teaching method, as well as increase in learner confidence; we found no studies of e-learning resources in rheumatology showing improved patient outcomes. Similarly, a 2012 systematic review of musculoskeletal clinical skills teaching found that none of the reviewed studies evaluated patient outcomes.[6]

There has been an increasing emphasis in the realm of educational scholarship on application of quality improvement and translational science[52] methodologies to learning intervention assessment. One study using a quality improvement approach found that an e-learning intervention for community rheumatologists improved their documentation of performance of 6 quality measures for rheumatoid arthritis care.[53] However, this study required funding support for chart review and physician time, which is often not feasible on an ongoing basis for many educational interventions. We identified no publications to date evaluating rheumatology e-learning resources from a translational science perspective.

SUMMARY

E-learning in rheumatology has expanded rapidly over the past 2 decades. A multitude of online resources has been developed, catering both to trainees and practicing health care providers, as opportunities to enhance clinical skills and knowledge of rheumatology and musculoskeletal medicine. Online platforms offer easy, flexible access and the ability to connect diverse learners and teachers to an unprecedented degree. In particular, the use of blended learning, where e-learning resources enhance face-to-face learning, is an exciting area for future inquiry. Additional research is required to optimize the role of e-learning in rheumatology and to validate impacts on learner education and patient care.

DISCLOSURE

The authors have no disclosures.

REFERENCES

1. Lewis KO, Cidon MJ, Seto TL, et al. Leveraging e-learning in medical education. Curr Probl Pediatr Adolesc Health Care 2014;44(6):150–63.
2. Ruiz JG, Mintzer MJ, Leipzig RM. The impact of E-learning in medical education. Acad Med 2006;81(3):207–12.
3. Cook DA. Web-based learning: pros, cons and controversies. Clin Med 2007; 7(1):37–42.
4. Ellaway R, Masters K. AMEE guide 32: e-Learning in medical education part 1: learning, teaching and assessment. Med Teach 2008;30(5):455–73.
5. Chodorow S. Educators must take the electronic revolution seriously. Acad Med 1996;71(3):221–6.
6. O'Dunn-Orto A, Hartling L, Campbell S, et al. Teaching musculoskeletal clinical skills to medical trainees and physicians: a Best Evidence in Medical Education systematic review of strategies and their effectiveness: BEME Guide No. 18. Med Teach 2012;34(2):93–102.
7. Lim SY, Bolster MB. Challenges in optimizing medical education for rheumatologists. Rheum Dis Clin North Am 2019;45(1):127–44.
8. Masters K, Ellaway R. e-Learning in medical education Guide 32 Part 2: Technology, management and design. Med Teach 2008;30(5):474–89.
9. Thomas PA, Kern DE, Hughes MT. Curriculum development for medical education: a six-step approach. 3rd edition. Baltimore (MD): Johns Hopkins University Press; 2016.
10. Miller GE. The assessment of clinical skills/competence/performance. Acad Med 1990;65(9 Suppl):S63–7.
11. Kirkpatrick DL, Kirkpatrick JD. Evaluating training programs: the four levels. 3rd edition. San Francisco (CA): Berrett-Koehler; 2006.
12. QSIN Institute. Quality and Safety Education for Nurses Institute. SQUIRE-EDU extension. 2017. Available at: http://qsen.org/squire-edu-v0-9/; http://www.squire-statement.org/index.cfm?fuseaction=document.viewDocument&documentid=59&documentFormatId=66&vDocLinkOrigin=1&CFID=9106588&CFTOKEN=cc0b4 a9e43bc798b-24D772C4-1C23-C8EB-805F99EF8CA44791I. Accessed March 6, 2019.
13. Kilian A, Upton LA, Battafarano DF, et al. Workforce trends in rheumatology. Rheum Dis Clin North Am 2019;45(1):13–26.
14. Global Alliance for Musculoskeletal Health. 2019. Available at: http://bjdonline.org/. Accessed April 7, 2019.
15. Association of American Medical Colleges. 2019. Available at: https://www.mededportal.org/. Accessed April 7, 2019.
16. Curran ML. Available at: https://ouchmyleg.northwestern.edu. Accessed April 7, 2019.
17. Curran M, Singh R. Development of a pediatric rheumatology education resource-sharing website: If you build it, will they come? Ann Rheum Dis 2015;74:407.
18. Vliet Vlieland TP, van den Ende CH, Alliot-Launois F, et al. Educational needs of health professionals working in rheumatology in Europe. RMD Open 2016;2(2): e000337.
19. Eular School of Rheumatology. EULAR online course on rheumatic diseases. Available at: https://esor.eular.org/theme/lc_eular/layout/enrol.php?id=10. Accessed March 6, 2019.

20. Beyer C, Ramiro S, Sivera F, et al. Educational needs and preferences of young European clinicians and physician researchers working in the field of rheumatology. RMD Open 2016;2(2):e000240.
21. University of South Wales. University of South Wales masters course in rheumatology. Available at: https://www.southwales.ac.uk/courses/msc-rheumatology-online-delivery/. Accessed March 6, 2019.
22. Rheumatology American College of Rheumatology. Educational activities. 2019. Available at: https://www.rheumatology.org/Learning-Center/Educational-Activities. Accessed April 7, 2019.
23. Rheumatology Research Foundation. Training and education awards. Available at: https://www.rheumresearch.org/education-and-training-awards#CSE. Accessed April 6, 2019.
24. Rheumatology Research Foundation. Clinician scholar educator award recipients. Available at: https://www.rheumresearch.org/clinician-scholar-educator-award-recipients. Accessed March 6, 2019.
25. Kissin EY, Niu J, Balint P, et al. Musculoskeletal ultrasound training and competency assessment program for rheumatology fellows. J Ultrasound Med 2013; 32(10):1735–43.
26. Ultrasound School of North American Rheumatologists. USSONAR training program. 2019. Available at: http://www.ussonar.org/training/overview/. Accessed April 6, 2019.
27. American Academy of Pediatrics. PREP rheumatology. 2019. Available at: https://shop.aap.org/2019-prep-rheumatology/. Accessed March 6, 2019.
28. Paediatric musculoskeletal matters. Available at: http://www.pmmonline.org/about-pmm. Accessed April 9, 2019.
29. Foster HE, Kay LJ, Friswell M, et al. Musculoskeletal screening examination (pGALS) for school-age children based on the adult GALS screen. Arthritis Rheum 2006;55(5):709–16.
30. Paediatric Musculoskeletal Matters. Paediatric gait, arms, leg, spine mobile application. Available at: http://www.pmmonline.org/page.aspx?id=342. Accessed April 9, 2019.
31. Haemel A, Kahl L, Callen J, et al. Supplementing dermatology physician resident education in vasculitis and autoimmune connective tissue disease: a prospective study of an online curriculum. JAMA Dermatol 2019;155(3):381–3.
32. UpToDate. 2019. Available at: https://www.uptodate.com/. Accessed April 7, 2019.
33. DynaMed. 2019. Available at: https://dynamed.com/home/. Accessed April 7, 2019.
34. Medscape. 2019. Available at: https://reference.medscape.com/. Accessed April 7, 2019.
35. StatPearls. 2019. Available at: https://www.statpearls.com/kb/index. Accessed April 7, 2019.
36. YouTube. 2019. Available at: https://www.youtube.com/. Accessed April 7, 2019.
37. Fischer J, Geurts J, Valderrabano V, et al. Educational quality of YouTube videos on knee arthrocentesis. J Clin Rheumatol 2013;19(7):373–6.
38. Apple Inc. 2019. Available at: https://www.apple.com/ios/app-store/. Accessed April 7, 2019.
39. Google. 2019. https://play.google.com/store/apps?hl=en_US. Accessed April 7, 2019.
40. Twitter I. 2019. Available at: https://twitter.com/. Accessed April 7, 2019.

41. Collins C. Twitter basics. Available at: https://www.slideshare.net/paulsufka/twitter-for-rheumatologists-45199060. Accessed April 7, 2019.
42. Collins C. 2019. Available at: https://twitter.com/RheumPearls. Accessed April 7, 2019.
43. Collins C, Sufka P, Bhana S, et al. 2019. Available at: https://twitter.com/RheumJC. Accessed April 9, 2019.
44. Wong G, Greenhalgh T, Pawson R. Internet-based medical education: a realist review of what works, for whom and in what circumstances. BMC Med Educ 2010;10:12.
45. Davis FD. Perceived usefulness, perceived ease of use, and user acceptance of information technology. MIS Q 1989;13:319–40.
46. Laurillard D. Rethinking University Teaching: a conversational framework for the effective use of learning technologies. 2nd edition. London: RoutledgeFalmer; 2002.
47. Walsh K. Mobile learning in medical education: review. Ethiop J Health Sci 2015; 25(4):363–6.
48. Vaona A, Banzi R, Kwag KH, et al. E-learning for health professionals. Cochrane Database Syst Rev 2018;(1):CD011736.
49. Sinclair P, Kable A, Levett-Jones T. The effectiveness of internet-based e-learning on clinician behavior and patient outcomes: a systematic review protocol. JBI Database System Rev Implement Rep 2015;13(1):52–64.
50. Prystowsky JB, Bordage G. An outcomes research perspective on medical education: the predominance of trainee assessment and satisfaction. Med Educ 2001;35(4):331–6.
51. Dauphinee WD. Educators must consider patient outcomes when assessing the impact of clinical training. Med Educ 2012;46(1):13–20.
52. McGaghie WC. Medical education research as translational science. Sci Transl Med 2010;2(19):19cm18.
53. Sapir T, Rusie E, Greene L, et al. Influence of continuing medical education on rheumatologists' performance on National Quality Measures for rheumatoid arthritis. Rheumatol Ther 2015;2(2):141–51.
54. American College of Rheumatology. Rheum2Learn. 2019. Available at: https://www.rheumatology.org/Learning-Center/Educational-Activities/Rheum2Learn. Accessed April 7, 2019.
55. Rheumatology ACo. Rheum4Science. 2019. Available at: https://www.rheumatology.org/Learning-Center/Educational-Activities/View/ID/881. Accessed April 7, 2019.
56. American College of Rheumatology. High impact rheumatology. 2019. Available at: https://www.rheumatology.org/Learning-Center/Educational-Activities/High-Impact-Rheumatology. Accessed April 7, 2019.
57. Versus arthritis. 2019. Available at: https://www.versusarthritis.org/about-arthritis/healthcare-professionals/. Accessed April 7, 2019.
58. Woodward A. A modular curriculum in pediatric rheuma-tology for residents, pediatric-ians and adult specialists. Available at: https://pediatrics.mc.vanderbilt.edu/interior.php?mid=10605. Accessed April 7. 2019.
59. D'Alessandro D, D'Alessandro M. Available at: Pediatriceducation.org https://pediatriceducation.org/casesbyspecialty/. Accessed April 9, 2019.
60. Cush JJ, Kavanaugh A, Stein CM. RheumaKnowledgy. Available at: http://www.rheumaknowledgy.com/. Accessed April 9, 2019.
61. Paediatric Musculoskeletal Matters International. Available at: http://www.pmmonline.org. Accessed April 9, 2019.

62. Univadis. Available at: ww.univadis.com/home/education?kw=keyword_rheumatology. Accessed April 9, 2019.
63. McGonagle D, Benjamin M. Enthesitis and enthesopathy. Available at: https://www.enthesis.info/. Accessed April 9, 2019.
64. The PIVOT project. Available at: https://www.the-pivot-project.org/. Accessed April 9, 2019.
65. Behrens E. JIA calculator. Available at: http://www.jra-research.org/JIAcalc/. Accessed April 9, 2019.
66. Introduction to paediatric musculoskeletal clinical skills - pGALS. Available at: https://cpd.ncl.ac.uk/courses/course-details/2. Accessed April 9, 2019.
67. Denman G, Barker A, Jandial S, et al. Paediatric musculoskeletal medicine in primary care. Available at: https://cpd.ncl.ac.uk/courses/course-details/5. Accessed April 9, 2019.
68. Emedicine pediatrics. Available at: https://emedicine.medscape.com/pediatrics_general. Accessed April 9, 2019.
69. Emedicine rheumatology. Available at: https://emedicine.medscape.com/rheumatology. Accessed April 9, 2019.
70. Papou A. Rheumatology mind map. Available at: http://rheumatologymindmap.com/. Accessed April 9, 2019.
71. Carmona R. RheumTutor. Available at: http://www.rheumtutor.com/. Accessed April 9. 2019.
72. Gillispie M, Muscal E, Rama J, et al. Pediatric rheumatology curriculum for the pediatrics resident: a case-based approach to learning. 2018. Available at: https://www.mededportal.org/publication/10767/. Accessed April 9, 2019.
73. Moroz A. Clinical reasoning workshop: cervical spine and shoulder disorders. 2017. Available at: https://www.mededportal.org/publication/10560/. Accessed April 9, 2019.
74. Scaperotti M, Gil N, Downs I, et al. Development and evaluation of a web-based dermatology teaching tool for preclinical medical students. 2017. Available at: https://www.mededportal.org/publication/10619/. Accessed April 9, 2019.
75. Gill P, MacPherson P, LeBlanc C, et al. PedsCases - a learning module for evaluation of a pediatric limp for medical students. 2010. Available at: https://www.mededportal.org/publication/7910/. Accessed April 9, 2019.
76. Rogers B, Ellsworth J. PedsCases: a learning module for an approach to juvenile idiopathic arthritis for medical students. 2010. Available at: https://www.mededportal.org/publication/10383/. Accessed April 9, 2019.
77. Averns H, Davidson L. Examination of the shoulder. 2013. Available at: https://www.mededportal.org/publication/9551/. Accessed April 9, 2019.
78. Akins R, Pema K. Sam rodilla - knee pain. 2012. Available at: https://www.mededportal.org/publication/9078/. Accessed.
79. Berger A, Sheth P, Bradley S. Low back pain ambulatory medicine cases. 2013. Available at: https://www.mededportal.org/publication/9565/. Accessed April 9, 2019.
80. Almoallim H, Alkatheeri A, Monjed A, et al. Structured oral examinations in internal medicine - case H. 2009. Available at: https://www.mededportal.org/publication/1120/. Accessed April 9, 2019.
81. Almoallim H, Kalantan D, Shabrawishi M, et al. Basic skills in musculoskeletal examination: hands-on training workshop. 2013. Available at: https://www.mededportal.org/publication/9398/. Accessed April 9, 2019.
82. Rubenstein B, Siddique F. Joint effusion workshop. 2016. Available at: https://www.mededportal.org/publication/10368/. Accessed April 9, 2019.

83. Bishop S, Kushinka J, Call S. Internal medicine clerkship team-based learning series: joint pain module. 2012. Available at: https://www.mededportal.org/publication/9147/. Accessed April 9, 2019.
84. Bishop S, Kushinka J, Call S. Internal medicine clerkship team-based learning series: back pain module. 2012. Available at: https://www.mededportal.org/publication/9153/. Accessed April 9, 2019.
85. Janssen SK, VanderMeulen SP, Brown D. Hands-on lightly embalmed cadaver lab for teaching knee aspiration/injection. 2012. Available at: https://www.mededportal.org/publication/9187/. Accessed April 9, 2019.
86. Peterson R. Pediatric rheumatology case-based e-learning modules. Available at: https://lpchrheum.moodlecloud.com/. Accessed February 20, 2019.
87. Macleod's Clinical Examination. Musculoskeletal gait arms legs spine exam video. Available at: https://www.youtube.com/watch?v=b8eSqR9Pu24. Accessed April 7, 2019.
88. Potter L. Geeky Medics. GALS examination (Gait, Arms, Legs, Spine) - OSCE Guide. Available at: https://www.youtube.com/watch?v=pClOlpzo-Jc. Accessed April 7, 2019.
89. Sherry D. Enthesitis examination video. Available at: http://www.youtube.com/watch?v=xtOLGlm1hhU. Accessed April 7, 2019.
90. Collins C. RheumPearls. Available at: www.rheumpearls.com https://twitter.com/RheumPearls. Accessed April 9, 2019.
91. O'Neill JM, Legault K. Essential Imaging in Rheumatology Clinical Case Challenge. Mobile application. Available at: https://apps.apple.com/ca/app/esimr-uncovering-the-hand-radiograph/id1160847576?mt=8. Accessed April 9, 2019.
92. O'Neill JM, Pritchett S. Essential Imaging in Rheumatology Uncovering the Hand Radiograph. Mobile application. Available at: https://apps.apple.com/ca/app/esimr-uncovering-the-hand-radiograph/id1160847576?mt=8. Accessed April 9, 2019.
93. O'Neill J, editor. Essential imaging in rheumatology. New York: Springer-Verlag; 2015.
94. iAnkylosingSpondylitis. Mobile application. Available at: https://apps.apple.com/us/app/iankylosingspondylitis/id414586259. Accessed April 9, 2019.
95. Rheumatology Advanced Vital Education (RAVE). Mobile application. Available at: https://apps.apple.com/us/app/rave-mobile/id505074662. Accessed April 9, 2019.
96. Gobert P. RheumaIQ. Mobile application. Available at: https://apps.apple.com/hu/app/rheuma-iq/id1267788382. Accessed April 9, 2019.
97. O'Neill JM, Russell C. Essential imaging in rheumatology unravelling spondyloarthropathy. Mobile application. Available at: https://apps.apple.com/ca/app/esimr-unravelling-spondyloarthropathy/id1160849005?mt=8. Accessed April 10, 2019.
98. @Point of Care Rheumatologic Diseases. Mobile application. Available at: https://apps.apple.com/us/app/rheumatologic-diseases-poc/id1251067402 Accessed April 9, 2019.
99. Collins C, Sufka P, Bhana S, et al. @RheumJC. rheumjc.com; Twitter feed #RheumJC. Available at: https://twitter.com/RheumJC. Accessed April 9. 2019.
100. CORE: Clinical Orthopedic Examination. Available at: http://clinicallyrelevant.com/core-clinical-orthopedic-exam/. Accessed April 9, 2019.

Modern Landscapes and Strategies for Learning Ultrasound in Rheumatology

Benjamin B. Widener, MD[a,b], Amy Cannella, MD, MS, RhMSUS[b,c], Linett Martirossian, MD[d], Eugene Y. Kissin, MD, RhMSUS[d,*]

KEYWORDS

- Ultrasound • Musculoskeletal ultrasound • Ultrasound in rheumatology • Education
- Competency assessment • Certification

KEY POINTS

- Ultrasound in rheumatology (RhUS) is evolving and many practitioners seek training in this imaging modality.
- Educational opportunities for RhUS exist in fellowship training and as a practicing clinician.
- Competency assessment for RhUS is not standardized in fellowship training, but certification examinations exist.

INTRODUCTION

Ultrasound (US) is a safe and reliable imaging modality that can dynamically assess multiple sites in one setting. The use of US at the point of care has changed the clinical landscape for the rheumatology sonographer, allowing point-of-care diagnosis, intervention and monitoring by the clinician trained in the pathology, diagnosis, and therapy of the patient's clinical presentation. US evaluation of rheumatic disease has evolved significantly over the past several decades. In 2012, the American College of Rheumatology (ACR) published a report on the reasonable use of musculoskeletal US (MSUS) in rheumatology clinical practice. An expert panel was developed to review the literature for the application of US to clinical scenarios.[1] Fourteen clinical

Disclosures: Dr B.B. Widener has no financial or commercial conflicts of interest. Dr A. Cannella is a board member and mentor for USSONAR. Dr L. Martirossian has no financial or commercial conflicts of interest. Dr E.Y. Kissin is a board member and mentor for USSONAR.
[a] 986270 Nebraska Medical Center, Omaha, NE 68198-6270, USA; [b] Omaha Veteran's Affairs Medical Center, Omaha, NE, USA; [c] UNMC Rheumatology, 986270 Nebraska Medical Center, Omaha, NE 68198-6270, USA; [d] Division of Rheumatology, Boston University Medical Center, 72 East Concord Street, Evans 506, Boston, MA, USA
* Corresponding author.
E-mail address: eukissin@bu.edu

scenarios achieved positive recommendations, and the level of evidence for each was graded from A to C. US has also been incorporated into recently revised classification criteria for gout and polymyalgia rheumatica (**Table 1**).[2,3] Initially limited to the musculoskeletal system, this important imaging modality is also used to image rheumatic disease pathology of the vasculature, salivary glands, and lungs. As indications for US in rheumatology (RhUS) expand and barriers to its adoption diminish, rheumatology practitioners at all levels will seek additional training and competency assessment.

EDUCATIONAL OPPORTUNITIES

Broadly, RhUS is learned in three ways:

1. Fellowship training
2. Mentored structured or nonstructured training
3. Self-directed, nonmentored training

Before RhUS training opportunities in fellowship, most practitioners were self-taught by attending courses, reading the literature, viewing on-line modules, and unsupervised practice. Self-directed learning requires a high degree of motivation, suffers from lack of feedback, and risks unidentified gaps or blind spots in training. Mentored training solves the problem of lack of feedback, although the quality of feedback is mentor dependent, and gaps in training also depend on the pedantic qualities of the individual mentor and learner. Curriculum-based, structured training helps avoid gaps in RhUS education and supports the mentor in providing a well-rounded education.

FELLOWSHIP-BASED TRAINING

In 2008, ACR member physicians, program directors, and fellows were surveyed to assess trends in MSUS by rheumatologists in the United States.[4] Thirty-three percent of fellowship program directors responded that 41% included MSUS in their training program. More than 63% of the responding ACR members (9% overall response rate) believed that MSUS should become a standard tool in rheumatology. In 2010

Table 1
Reasons for a rheumatologist to use ultrasound

Region Specific	Disease Specific	Guidance
Evaluation of peripheral articular pain or swelling	Evaluation of asymptomatic joints in patients with inflammatory arthritis for subclinical inflammation	For guidance of needle placement into articular and periarticular aspiration and injection
Evaluation of mechanical shoulder disorder		
Evaluation of mechanical hip disorder	Evaluation of disease activity and damage in peripheral joints of patients with inflammatory arthritis	For guidance of synovial biopsy
Evaluation of soft tissue disorders affecting tendons and ligaments	Evaluation for suspected enthesitis	
Evaluation of peripheral nerve entrapment	Evaluation of suspected Sjögren disease of the salivary glands	
	Evaluation of suspected crystal arthritis	
	Evaluation of suspected polymyalgia rheumatica	

and 2013, the ACR continued to survey program directors regarding training in MSUS, which showed increasing trends in US education during fellowship.[5,6] A 2009 survey assessed implementation of MSUS during fellowship across 31 European countries.[7] MSUS was required in seven countries (22.6%), optional or recommended in 11 (35.5%), and not included in 13 (42%). Only six (19.4%) had competency assessment as part of the curriculum. It is likely that similar to American training programs, these numbers will have increased in the past decade.

In 2017, two surveys were sent to American rheumatology fellowship programs, with a response rate of 96% of program directors.[8] This survey clearly demonstrated that RhUS education has evolved such that 94% of fellowship programs offer training in RhUS, and there is a need for a formalized yet optional fellowship curriculum. Subsequently, the ACR endorsed the development of an RhUS curriculum, which was completed in 2019.[9] This curriculum identifies the goals and objectives for an educational RhUS program, including supplements for pediatrics, scanning guides, documentation templates, and toolboxes for activities and assessments. Curricular milestones, spanning a 12-month period, were developed to assist program directors in assessing the progression of a fellow through an institutional-specific training program. Although there has been a marked increase in educational opportunities during fellowship, competency in RhUS is not currently a requirement for rheumatology training in the United States or most European countries,[10–12] and no competency assessment tools were included as part of this curriculum.

The use of MSUS is prevalent in other musculoskeletal medicine specialties in the United States. Given the increasing clinical acceptance and available educational modalities, specialty-specific curriculum and training are being established and implemented. A 2016 survey asked program directors from the following four specialties to assess US training (survey response rate): (1) physical medicine and rehabilitation (PM&R) (23%), (2) rheumatology (28%), (3) radiology (25%), and (4) sports medicine (33%). One hundred percent of PM&R, 90% of rheumatology, 88% of sports medicine, and 65% of radiology program directors reported that they teach MSUS, and those not teaching plan to implement MSUS training within the next 5 years.[13] Based on other survey data of PM&R residencies, 97% of respondents report exposure to MSUS and 44% have a formal curriculum.[14] In fact, MSUS training is now an ACGME (The Accreditation Council for Graduate Medical Education) requirement of PM&R residency programs.[15]

The mechanisms by which clinical US skills are taught in formal training programs are broad and tend to include reading assignments; multimedia didactics; hands-on scanning; outside courses; and human, simulator, and cadaveric models.[12,13,16–18] In a small study, 15 orthopedic surgery residents were assessed on their ability to identify and quantify three ankle tendons after receiving education from a multimedia educational tutorial and showed a 90% to 94.8% success rate.[19] Simulation is also a frequently and effectively deployed modality for teaching a variety of procedures in internal medicine.[20] Based on small trials comparing point-of-care US training/education methods, structured and multimodal training is effective for teaching bedside US in other disciplines, such as critical care and emergency medicine.[21] These methods of training should be applicable to RhUS training.

MENTOR-BASED TRAINING

Before formalized fellowship training, the Ultrasound School of North American Rheumatologists (USSONAR) was formed by a group of self-trained and mentor-trained rheumatologists to help mitigate the deficiency of local mentors and lack of

RhUS curricular training. In 2008, the group collaborated to create an 8-month curriculum of reading materials, online assignments, and a hands-on workshop. World Wide Web–based mentoring through US study review and feedback is central to the USSONAR teaching program, such that participants without local mentors can still receive a comprehensive education in RhUS. Each participant is assessed though written and practical scanning examination at the completion of the program.

SELF-DIRECTED, NONMENTORED TRAINING

Multiple self-directed learning opportunities exist for RhUS, irrespective of the chosen educational path. Available resources to guide rheumatology sonographers include text books, online Internet-based resources (Web sites, tutorials, videos, journals), and continuing education courses, each having particular advantages and disadvantages. There are several available textbooks for learning the technical, anatomic, and procedural aspects of RhUS (**Box 1**).[18] These textbooks range in their depth and breadth, and allow for self-directed study and knowledge acquisition, but cannot provide the real-time skills needed for actual RhUS practice, the latter of which is best obtained by using multiple modalities to optimize the knowledge of anatomy, US technology, hands-on scanning skills, and practical applications.

Online resources include several educational modalities from a broad array of organizations that include university and society Web sites, which can effectively teach US (**Table 2**).[18] In a small study of radiology residents/fellows with limited abdominal US experience, they were able to objectively improve their skills and raise their own perceived confidence by using a World Wide Web–based video created for education.[22] In addition, YouTube contains many free instructional videos from a wide range of sources on RhUS techniques. In a review of available non-RhUS but point-of-care US videos relative to internal medicine, most were well regarded in terms of their educational value, but noted a lack of available safety-related information.[23] Although videos are free and open access, they are not necessarily peer-reviewed, and the quality, intent, and accuracy of information may vary.

There are many independently available resources to advance education and skills in RhUS, but hands-on experience is an absolute requirement. Other studies

---

Box 1
List of textbooks

- Bruyn GA, Schmidt WA. *Introductory guide to musculoskeletal ultrasound for the rheumatologist.* Houten (The Netherlands): Bohn Stafleu van Loghum; 2005.

- Bianchi S, Martinoli C. *Ultrasound of the musculoskeletal system.* Berlin: Springer; 2007.

- Jacobson J. *Fundamentals of musculoskeletal ultrasound.* Philadelphia: Saunders; 2012.

- Wakefield RJ, D'Agostino MA. *Essential applications of musculoskeletal ultrasound in rheumatology.* Philadelphia: Saunders Elsevier; 2010.

- Schuenke M, Schulte E, Schumacher U. *General anatomy and musculoskeletal system (THIEME Atlas of Anatomy).* New York: Thieme; 2010.

- Kohler M. *Musculoskeletal ultrasound in rheumatology review.* Switzerland: Springer International Publishing; 2016.

Adapted from Cannella AC, Kissin EY, Torralba KD, et al. Evolution of musculoskeletal ultrasound in the United States: implementation and practice in rheumatology. Arthritis Care Res (Hoboken) 2014;66(1):11; with permission.

Table 2
Ultrasound resources

Site	A	B	C	D	E	F
AIUM: www.AIUM.org	X			X		
University of Michigan: https://www.med.umich.edu/radiology/mskus/index.html	X			X		
ESSR: https://www.essr.org/subcommittees/ultrasound/	X					
USSONAR: www.ussonar.org	X	X	X	X		
ACR certification information: https://www.rheumatology.org/Learning-Center/RhMSUS-Certification			X	X		
ACR Image bank: http://images.rheumatology.org/					X	
EULAR: www.eular.org		X		X		
EULAR Image Data Bank: https://www.eular.org/eular_imaging_library_portal.cfm#					X	
ARDMS: www.ardms.org			X			
EFSUMB: www.efsumb.org						X
MedEdPortal: www.mededportal.org	X				X	X

A, Online region-based tutorial, protocols, technical guidelines; B, Online training program with certification; C, Certification program through written examination; D, On-site courses and/or workshops; E, Online pictorial essays, anatomy-ultrasound correlation; F, Competency-based assessments and evaluation tools and training recommendations.

Abbreviations: AIUM, American Institute of Ultrasound in Medicine; ARDMS, American Registry for Diagnostic Sonography; EFSUMB, European Federation of Societies for Ultrasound in Medicine and Biology; ESSR, European Society of Musculoskeletal Radiology; EULAR, European League Against Rheumatism.

Adapted from Cannella AC, Kissin EY, Torralba KD, et al. Evolution of musculoskeletal ultrasound in the United States: implementation and practice in rheumatology. Arthritis Care Res (Hoboken) 2014;66(1):11; with permission.

note that training in one area of US may lead to overconfidence in another area, and the role of supervised and qualified training cannot be overstated.[21,24] Although this supervision or mentoring may not be locally available for all practitioners desiring to learn RhUS, many 2- or 3-day continuing education courses exist and can provide a surrogate for supervision. The ACR, European League Against Rheumatism, USSONAR, and other private courses are well attended and can provide education for the beginner, intermediate, and advanced sonographer.[18] Clinicians can also pay for access to the curriculum, online modules, and scanning guides of USSONAR. Other available resources include the American Institute of Ultrasound in Medicine, which provides a variety of online lectures and educational events, including hands-on courses. The American Institute of Ultrasound in Medicine considers these courses and materials to be appropriate for sonographers, physicians, and other professionals involved in the assessment and treatment of patients with musculoskeletal disorders. These and other privately available courses provide considerable educational opportunity for the fellow in training and the practicing clinician.

The increasing use and acceptance of US in medical practice among a variety of specialties is being bolstered by increasing fellowship training opportunities and a multitude of available educational resources aimed at practicing clinicians. There remain challenges to operationalizing the ideal training curriculum for fellowship and practicing clinicians, but fortunately there exists a wide array of resources to improve and optimize this clinical skillset.

IMPLEMENTING ULTRASOUND IN RHEUMATOLOGY

The practicing rheumatologist could first focus on the US techniques that are easy to learn and highly applicable to clinical problem solving. With more experience, the sonographer may then incorporate more challenging techniques. Following this strategy to establish a sequence of learning may lead to greater learner satisfaction and motivation to continue. In addition to avoiding blind spots within the training, RhUS curricula can assist the learner in identification of a knowledge base necessary to start the practice of RhUS and pass a competency examination.

Most RhUS educational curriculums include learning when and why to perform US assessment, how to perform the assessment, and how to interpret and report the assessment. Some work has also been aimed at distinguishing core from intermediate and advanced RhUS knowledge and skill. Core has been described as identification of synovial effusion, synovial hypertrophy, tenosynovitis, erosion, osteophyte, bursitis, and cysts. The intermediate level requires identification of tendinopathy, tendon tear and enthesitis, and the use of US for guided procedures. The advanced level includes using US for monitoring of disease activity, nerve entrapment, muscle and ligament injury, and calcification.[25] However, this does not necessarily mean that advanced level training is more difficult to achieve than core level.

ATTAINING COMPETENCY

Although no standardized definition of competency exists for RhUS, over time and with training, the novice sonographer may progressively attain competency when compared with expert sonographers. For example, identification of synovial hypertrophy is considered a core skill, but in a study of knee osteoarthritis, interreader agreement for synovial hypertrophy (comparing expert and novice sonographers) was only 0.4.[26] However, evaluation of nerve entrapment (an advanced training component) yielded excellent interclass correlation between an expert and novice sonographer with just 2 months (30 studies) of experience ($r = 0.95$).[27]

Based on a competency definition of good interreader reliability between the learner and expert sonographer, it is easier to attain competency for assessment of a Baker cyst or knee effusion than for assessment of synovial hypertrophy or cartilage thinning in the knee.[26] Arguably, the former is more clinically useful.

Similarly, the ability to diagnose compressive neuropathy without the need for nerve conduction studies adds substantial value to clinical practice. After 2 days of training, 19 novice sonographers and were able to determine the cross-sectional area of a median nerve to within 1 mm of the value determined by an expert sonographer.[28] In contrast, assessing rheumatoid arthritis by US seems to be more challenging. A study comparing grayscale synovial hypertrophy assessment in the wrist and metacarpal-phalangeal joints in patients with rheumatoid arthritis between novice sonographers ($\leq$100 scans per year) and experienced sonographers ($\geq$100 scans per year), found good interrater reliability (0.64) for the experienced sonographers but poor reliability (0.12) by novice sonographers.[29] The authors also found a substantial difference between experienced and novice sonographers for detecting erosions (0.41 vs 0.12), and for identification of Doppler signal (0.63 vs 0.0). Furthermore, the difference in US results between the novice and experienced sonographer was magnified when the scanning was performed with a low-quality machine. This suggests that it is easier to achieve technical competence with higher quality equipment.

Shoulder sonography is another frequent stumbling block for novices because of (1) the multiple views required for complete assessment of the region, (2) the need for frequent machine setting adjustments between views, and (3) the lower familiarity with the anatomy of the shoulder among rheumatologists when compared with the wrist and hand. However, after a 4-day course in MSUS, an orthopedic surgeon was able to correctly identify 20 out of 26 rotator cuffs with full-thickness tears. In this study, it should be noted that the evaluations were performed as part of daily practice during which 350 consecutive shoulders were scanned, and there was likely improvement in technical ability that occurred throughout the duration of the study. Unfortunately, the sequence for the missed tears among the 350 total scans was not reported. Finally, partial-thickness tears were likely more problematic because six out of seven were missed.[30] It is not clear how critical finding partial-thickness tears is to a rheumatologist.

Evaluation for gouty arthritis can also require a moderate amount of training. After 2 to 3 months of general MSUS training, an additional 5 days of instruction (4 hours per day) was needed to maximize agreement with an MSUS expert for detection of erosion or bursitis. Moreover, 7 days were required to achieve similar results for tendon inflammation, double contour sign, or intra-articular tophi.[31]

By comparison, training for US-guided needle placement may require less time. After 70 minutes of didactics and 140 minutes of practical instruction with a 1:3 instructor to student ratio, and using phantom blocks and mannequin arms for training, 74% of students were able to pass the standardized examination of US-guided venipuncture.[32] A study of 15 trainees learning to perform sciatic nerve block under US guidance, with feedback given between each attempt on a cadaveric model, found that on average 28 (range, 25–29) trials were required to achieve competency (defined as 90% chance of successful needle placement).[33] For arthrocentesis, a fellow with 3 months of general MSUS training along with 36 additional US-guided joint injections, was able to achieve accurate needle placement into joints including the shoulders, knees, elbows, wrists, and ankles 83% of the time (ranging from 63% to 91% depending on the joint region). This was significantly greater than the 66% accuracy achieved by experienced rheumatologists (**Fig. 1**).[34]

Overall, one study found that performing more than five scans per week for 6 months or having more than 1 year of MSUS training resulted in a high likelihood of passing an MSUS competency assessment.[35] A separate study showed that after an 8-month

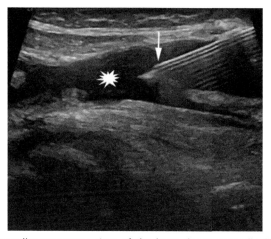

Fig. 1. This suprapatellar transverse view of the knee shows a needle (*arrow*) within the pocket of fluid (*star*) in the suprapatellar recess. This knee aspiration was performed by a rheumatology fellow.

training period with an average of 41 comprehensive MSUS studies performed and evaluated, 90% of participants were able to interpret US images of basic joint and soft tissue pathology and obtain standard US images of normal joint regions similar to experts in MSUS.[36] Additionally, mentored feedback on the submitted studies improved practical scanning results, but not necessarily US image interpretation results. Finally, rheumatology sonographers with 6 to 23 years of US experience (5000–50,000 scans) were compared with those with 2 to 4 years of US experience (250–1500 scans), and no differences in diagnostic accuracy were found. Both groups had an accuracy rate of 73% with reliability of 0.41.[37] Interrater reliability for tissue-specific pathology was slightly higher for the more experienced examiners at 0.43 as compared with 0.34 for the less experienced group ($P = .001$).

CERTIFICATION EXAMINATIONS

One can thus appreciate how RhUS competency may be attained in a modular fashion over a period of 1 to 2 years, especially if mentoring is available. However, because acquisition of RhUS skill is highly dependent on factors intrinsic to the learner, such as aptitude and motivation, and extrinsic to the learner, such as access to and quality of equipment, mentor availability, mentor teaching prowess, and curricular design, training time–based establishment of competency is not reliable. Instead, certification examinations may be used to ascertain that a minimal level of competence has been achieved. There are currently two options in the United States for RhUS certification examination. One examination is offered by the ACR and has been developed by rheumatologists for rheumatologists. It has a focus on the use of US for diagnosis and monitoring of rheumatic diseases.[37] To qualify for this multiple choice–based examination the candidate must complete at least 150 RhUS studies within the preceding 3 years and have attained at least 24 hours of continuing medical education credit in RhUS with at least 14 of the credits coming from a hands-on RhUS course. The second option is available through the Alliance for Physician Certification and Advancement, and has been created by a mixture of specialties. It has an emphasis on sports medicine and PM&R content. To qualify for this written examination, the candidate must submit a third-party attestation of having completed at least 150 studies in the preceding 3 years, but without any continuing medical education credit requirement. Especially for rheumatologist who acquire RhUS through self-directed learning outside of fellowship training, certification through one of these organizations helps ensure accountability to the public and to the insurance providers. Faculty who design and implement curricula aimed at achievement of RhUS competence, or develop the certification examinations for assessment of RhUS competence, are rewarded by their personal growth of reputation among the RhUS community, and more importantly, the reputation growth of the RhUS community as a whole in the eyes of the public.

SUMMARY

The interest in RhUS has grown over the past two decades, to a point where most fellowship programs offer RhUS training. Additional training opportunities through live and World Wide Web–based courses have emerged, as have the opportunities for certification in RhUS. Although clinicians in practice find a wide array of resources available for self-directed education in RUS, a consensus-based and publicly available training curriculum can further enhance and standardize the learning. Currently available research data provide preliminary evidence for standardizing RhUS training requirements. Specifically, the amount of training necessary to develop competence in the various applications can now be estimated. The past decade has provided some responses to previous RhUS learning barriers, which include equipment cost, lack of mentorship, and bureaucracy based resistance: (1) new equipment manufacturers and advances in technology have resulted in substantially lower equipment cost, (2) there are now more than 400 rheumatologists in the United States trained in RhUS and World Wide Web–based mentorship is available, and (3) the availability of RhUS certification provides rheumatologists with a means to prove their competence to the hospital and insurance managers.

ACKNOWLEDGMENTS

The authors acknowledge Teresa Hartman (University of Nebraska Medical Center McGoogan Library of Medicine) for her significant contributions in our literature review and Amrita Bath, MBBS (Fellow, University of Nebraska Medical Center) for the ultrasound image.

REFERENCES

1. McAlindon T, Kissin E, Nazarian L, et al. American College of Rheumatology report on reasonable use of musculoskeletal ultrasonography in rheumatology clinical practice. Arthritis Care Res (Hoboken) 2012;64:1625–40.
2. Neogi T, Jansen TL, Dalbeth N, et al. Gout classification criteria: an American College of Rheumatology/European League Against Rheumatism collaborative initiative. Ann Rheum Dis 2015;74:1789–98.
3. Dasgupta B, Cimmino MA, Kremers HM, et al. Provisional classification criteria for polymyalgia rheumatica: a European League Against Rheumatism/American College of Rheumatology collaborative initiative. Arthritis Rheum 2012;64:943–54.
4. Samuels J, Abramson SB, Kaeley GS. The use of musculoskeletal ultrasound by rheumatologists in the United States. Bull NYU Hosp Jt Dis 2010;68:292–8.
5. Force WMaRACoRMCT. 2010 Musculoskeletal ultrasound research: training directors survey (Nov 23-Dec 10, 2010). 2010.
6. Higgs J. American College of rheumatology 2013 program director survey in musculoskeletal ultrasound. American College of Rheumatology Program Directors Meeting. Chicago, IL, March 16, 2013.
7. Naredo E, D'Agostino M, Conaghan P, et al. Current state of musculoskeletal ultrasound training and implementation in Europe: results of a survey of experts and scientific societies. Rheumatology 2010;49:2438–43.
8. Torralba KD, Cannella AC, Kissin EY, et al. Musculoskeletal ultrasound instruction in adult rheumatology fellowship programs. Arthritis Care Res (Hoboken) 2017. [Epub ahead of print].
9. Cannella AC, Kissin EY, Torralba KD, et al. 2019 Rheumatologic ultrasound curriculum supplement to the American College of Rheumatology 2015 core curriculum outline. Atlanta (GA): American College of Rheumatology Program Directors Meeting. Chicago, IL, March 9, 2019.
10. Bolster M, Brown C, Criscione-Schreiber L, et al. Core curriculum outline for rheumatology fellowship programs updated June 2015. Atlanta, GA: American College of Rheumatology; 2015.
11. Training requirements for the specialty of rheumatology: European standards of postgraduate medical specialist training. 2014. Available at: https://www.uems.eu/. Accessed February 22, 2019.
12. Torralba KD. Musculoskeletal ultrasound instruction in adult rheumatology fellowship programs. Arthritis Care Res (Hoboken) 2010. [Epub ahead of print].

13. Berko NS, Goldberg-Stein S, Thornhill BA, et al. Survey of current trends in post-graduate musculoskeletal ultrasound education in the United States. Skeletal Radiol 2016;45:475–82.

14. Siddiqui IJ, Luz J, Borg-Stein J, et al. The current state of musculoskeletal ultrasound education in physical medicine and rehabilitation residency programs; 26690020. PM R 2016;8:660–6.

15. Luz J, Siddiqui I, Jain NB, et al. Resident-perceived benefit of a diagnostic and interventional musculoskeletal ultrasound curriculum: a multifaceted approach using independent study, peer teaching, and interdisciplinary collaboration; 26098924. Am J Phys Med Rehabil 2015;94:1095–103.

16. Berko NS, Le JN, Thornhill BA, et al. Design and validation of a peer-teacher-based musculoskeletal ultrasound curriculum. Acad Radiol 2018;26(5):701–6.

17. Eroglu O, Coskun F. Medical students' knowledge of ultrasonography: effects of a simulation-based ultrasound training program; 30374368. Pan Afr Med J 2018;30.

18. Cannella AC, Kissin EY, Torralba KD, et al. Evolution of musculoskeletal ultrasound in the United States: implementation and practice in rheumatology. Arthritis Care Res 2014;66:7–13.

19. Piposar JR, Easley M, Nunley JA, et al. Musculoskeletal ultrasound education: orthopaedic resident ability following a multimedia tutorial. J Surg Orthop Adv 2015; 24:64–8.

20. Sacks CA, Alba GA, Miloslavsky EM. The evolution of procedural competency in internal medicine training; 29059281. JAMA Intern Med 2017;177:1713–4.

21. Turner EE, Fox JC, Rosen M, et al. Implementation and assessment of a curriculum for bedside ultrasound training. J Ultrasound Med 2015;34:823–8.

22. Back SJ, Darge K, Bedoya MA, et al. Ultrasound tutorials in under 10 minutes: experience and results; 27276225. AJR Am J Roentgenol 2016;207:653–60.

23. Khandelwal A, Devine LA, Otremba M. Quality of widely available video instructional materials for point-of-care ultrasound-guided procedure training in internal medicine; 28370388. J Ultrasound Med 2017;36:1445–52.

24. Taggart A, Filipucci E, Wright G, et al. e. Musculoskeletal ultrasound training in rheumatology: the Belfast experience. Rheumatology 2006;45:102–5.

25. Brown AK, Roberts TE, O'Connor PJ, et al. The development of an evidence-based educational framework to facilitate the training of competent rheumatologist ultrasonographers; 17264091. Rheumatology 2007;46:391–7.

26. Iagnocco A, Perricone C, Scirocco C, et al. The interobserver reliability of ultrasound in knee osteoarthritis. Rheumatology (Oxford) 2012;51:2013–9.

27. Garcia-Santibanez R, Dietz AR, Bucelli RC, et al. Nerve ultrasound reliability of upper limbs: effects of examiner training. Muscle Nerve 2018;57:189–92.

28. Ozcakar L, Palamar D, Carl AB, et al. Precision of novice sonographers concerning median nerve and Achilles tendon measurements. Am J Phys Med Rehabil 2011;90:913–6.

29. Brulhart L, Ziswiler HR, Tamborrini G, et al. The importance of sonographer experience and machine quality with regards to the role of musculoskeletal ultrasound in routine care of rheumatoid arthritis patients. Clin Exp Rheumatol 2015;33: 98–101.

30. Moosmayer S, Smith HJ. Diagnostic ultrasound of the shoulder–a method for experts only? Results from an orthopedic surgeon with relative inexpensive compared to operative findings. Acta Orthop 2005;76:503–8.

31. Gutierrez M, Di Geso L, Rovisco J, et al. Ultrasound learning curve in gout: a disease-oriented training program. Arthritis Care Res (Hoboken) 2013;65: 1265–74.
32. McKay GFM, Weerasinghe A. Can we successfully teach novice junior doctors basic interventional ultrasound in a single focused training session? Postgrad Med J 2018;94:259–62.
33. Chen XX, Trivedi V, AlSaflan AA, et al. Ultrasound-guided regional anesthesia simulation training: a systematic review. Reg Anesth Pain Med 2017;42:741–50.
34. Cunnington J. A randomized, double-blind, controlled study of ultrasound-guided corticosteroid injection into the joint of patients with inflammatory arthritis. Arthritis Rheum 2010;62:1862–9.
35. Filippucci E, Meenagh G, Ciapetti A, et al. E-learning in ultrasonography: a web-based approach. Ann Rheum Dis 2007;66:962–5.
36. Kissin EY, Niu J, Balint P, et al. Musculoskeletal ultrasound training and competency assessment program for rheumatology fellows. J Ultrasound Med 2013; 32:1735–43.
37. Kissin EY, Nishio J, Yang M, et al. Self-directed learning of basic musculoskeletal ultrasound among rheumatologists in the United States. Arthritis Care Res (Hoboken) 2010;62:155–60.

Enhancing the Inpatient Consultation Learning Environment to Optimize Teaching and Learning

Naomi Serling-Boyd, MD, Eli M. Miloslavsky, MD*

KEYWORDS

- Inpatient consultation • Learning environment • Fellow as teacher • Fellow
- Resident

KEY POINTS

- Consult volume across specialties has been increasing over time in academic medical centers.
- Teaching in the setting of consultation is valued by both fellows and primary teams and may have broad-reaching positive effects.
- There are multiple barriers to effective consult interactions, which include workload, experience, lack of familiarity between teams, and hospital systems, among others.
- Interventions directed at improving the quality of consultation requests and enhancing fellows' teaching skills may enhance consult interactions between primary teams and subspecialties.

INTRODUCTION

Subspecialty consultation is becoming an increasingly used resource in inpatient medicine. An analysis of Medicare data suggests that an average Medicare patient receives 2.6 consults per admission, and a recent study of medicine hospitalists suggested that more than half request multiple consultations daily.[1,2] Several studies, including unpublished data from our center, suggest that the number of inpatient consultations has been steadily increasing over time.[3,4]

In addition to providing clinical care, studies have shown that an optimal consult interaction includes both effective communication with, and teaching directed to,

Disclosure: The authors have nothing to disclose.
Division of Rheumatology, Allergy and Immunology, Department of Medicine, Massachusetts General Hospital, Harvard Medical School, 55 Fruit Street, Bulfinch 165, Boston, MA 02114, USA
* Corresponding author.
E-mail address: emiloslavsky@mgh.harvard.edu

Rheum Dis Clin N Am 46 (2020) 73–83
https://doi.org/10.1016/j.rdc.2019.09.003
0889-857X/20/© 2019 Elsevier Inc. All rights reserved.
rheumatic.theclinics.com

the team requesting consultation.[5,6] Research from our group suggests that both housestaff and hospitalist primary teams have a strong desire to learn and that fellows have a strong desire to teach in the setting of inpatient consultation.[2,7,8] Furthermore, fellow teaching has been identified as part of the core competencies by the Accreditation Council for Graduate Medical Education (ACGME).[9] An effective teaching interaction during consultation has many potential benefits. Effective consults that include teaching can help optimize communication between teams, empower the primary team to provide effective care, and avoid miscommunication.[10] In addition, given the anticipated workforce shortage within rheumatology, consultation may be an important tool to recruit residents to our specialty. Kolasinski and colleagues[11] have demonstrated that most rheumatology fellows make the decision to pursue rheumatology during residency, and a study by Horn and colleagues[12] suggested that subspecialty fellows have an impact on the career choice of internal medicine residents. Therefore, fellow teaching and establishing good rapport with residents during inpatient consultation may help recruit trainees to our specialty because residents have the greatest exposure to rheumatology fellows in this setting.[13]

Given the importance and the potential positive effects of teaching and effective communication during consultation, several studies have sought to explore the primary team-consultant interaction. Herein we will explore what is known about the barriers to providing effective teaching during consultation and interventions that enhance the consult interaction. This literature has the potential to empower fellows to provide more effective consultation and faculty to explore and enhance the complex inpatient learning environment.

BARRIERS TO EFFECTIVE TEACHING DURING CONSULTATION

Despite the fact that teaching during consultation has many potential benefits and is desired by both residents and fellows, our previous work suggests that fellows are an underused teaching resource.[14,15] This may be because the primary team-consultant interaction is an example of situated learning[16] taking place in the academic medical center environment, which presents many potential barriers to effective consultation and an optimal learning environment. These factors can be broadly divided into interpersonal and systems issues (**Box 1**).

Box 1
Barriers to effective consultation

Interpersonal barriers

- Perceptions of primary teams and fellows
- "Pushback" on consult requests from fellows
- Willingness of primary teams to engage fellows in teaching

Systems barriers

- Inexperience
- Lack of familiarity between teams
- Workload
- Acclimating to a new hospital
- Quality of the consult request
- Fellows' teaching skills

Workload and Burnout

Fellows are likely being asked to do more than ever before. Fellows serve multiple roles within their divisions, including providing clinical care to both inpatients and outpatients, contributing to the research enterprise and teaching trainees who rotate in their subspecialty. Although there are no studies specifically addressing fellow workload, the increase in overall consultation volume without a concomitant expansion of fellowship positions, coupled with increasing patient complexity, suggest that fellow workload has likely been expanding. Consequences of increased workload may include less time for teaching, increased pushback on consult requests (defined as perceived resistance to perform consultation), higher rates of burnout, and potential detriments to patient care. Similarly, medicine hospitalists cited workload as a critical factor in their ability to learn from consultants.[2] In addition, when the fellow is finishing rounds later in the day, the ability to relay the recommendations in person to the primary team, which is a key factor to effective teaching, may be impaired.

Rates of burnout among residents and fellows remain high, and higher than medical students, practicing physicians in their early careers, as well as age-matched controls in other professions.[16] Approximately half of residents and fellows experience emotional exhaustion and high levels of depersonalization.[17] Another study looking at burnout among oncology fellows showed that feelings of emotional exhaustion and depersonalization actually increased from the beginning to the end of the first year of fellowship, and that perceived personal accomplishment decreased throughout the year, potentially demonstrating a link between high workload and burnout.[18] The concomitant and interrelated pressures of increasing workload and burnout may contribute significantly to both patient care and the learning environment during inpatient consultation. In addition, uncertainty, which is prevalent within rheumatology, may affect student, resident, and fellow interactions because uncertainty has been associated with increased psychological distress.[19,20] An unsupportive learning environment, which may also include institutional biases and insufficient resources for reflective practice, may adversely affect fellow personal and professional growth. This is of particular importance given that fellows are the future leaders of our field.

Interpersonal Barriers to Teaching During Consultation

Interpersonal factors impeding teaching during consultation include fellow pushback, residents' willingness to engage in teaching interactions, as well as perceptions and expectations of both the requesting and consulting teams.[8]

Fellow pushback on primary team consult requests, defined as communicating a perceived reluctance to perform the consultation, represents a critical barrier to teaching during consultation. It is important to note that residents and fellows may perceive pushback differently.[8] For example, a fellow's attempt to clarify the consult question may be perceived by the resident as an attempt to push back against the consult. However, that perception is in itself important, because such perceptions diminish the possibility that an effective teaching interaction occurs between that resident and fellow. Because the resident-fellow teaching interaction is often initiated by the resident (eg, by asking the fellow a question to elicit teaching), perceived or real fellow pushback is a major detriment to residents initiating the teaching interaction.[8] Furthermore, our group has found that residents often perceive that fellows are too busy to teach and that fellows often perceive that residents are too busy to learn during inpatient consultation.[8]

Other Systems Barriers to Teaching During Consultation

Multiple barriers to effective consultation arise as a result of hospital system factors. These include issues surrounding the consultation request, giving recommendations to the team, and the learning environment during inpatient consultation. The quality of the consult request can vary significantly by the level of training of the provider as well as their knowledge of the individual patient. Primary team structure can influence the quality of the consult request and also the fellow's ability to give in-person recommendations and teaching; for example, if the intern or resident calling the consult did not admit the patient, they may not be able to provide as much context. In addition, if the fellow finishes rounding late in the day and the primary provider has signed out to a covering intern, this person may not be as interested or have as much time to delve deeper into the case.[8] Furthermore, the consultant's knowledge of hospital systems is a common barrier. For example, not knowing where the resident work rooms are located or when the team signs out can make it difficult for the fellow to find the primary team and have an in-person discussion.

Familiarity (or the lack thereof) between residents and fellows has a significant effect on resident-fellow interactions. Several studies have demonstrated that familiarity between the resident and fellow, as well as the trust that familiarity helps create, are critical factors that enhance the consultation relationship.[2,8,21] Conversely, lack of familiarity can be a significant barrier, leading to pushback, less desire to teach on the part of the fellow, or less willingness to engage the fellow in teaching on the part of the resident.

Several barriers play a particularly important role during phases that are critical to fellows' professional identity formation, such as the beginning of fellowship.[22] Acclimating to a new hospital and learning the hospital system is a major impediment that can also exacerbate the barriers described above. In addition, toward the beginning of the academic year, fellows may be hesitant to give recommendations or provide teaching before discussing the case with the attending.[23] For example, for a complex patient with a fever of unknown origin, the fellow may be hesitant to lead the team down a particular diagnostic road without first fully discussing the case with an attending, even though simply leading the team through their initial thought process would be a great educational experience for both parties. By the time the patient is staffed there may be limited time or opportunity to teach the primary team. Barriers such as these are particularly important to address because they affect professional identity formation, including fellows' approach to primary team interactions. Setting their approach to consultation early in the year may prevent fellows from spending more time teaching as they gain confidence and experience.

Finally, fellows' teaching skills may be an additional barrier.[8] Although most fellows feel confident in their ability to teach, teaching in the setting of consultation poses significant challenges that differ from their previous teaching experiences.[7] For example, in contrast to teaching their team as a senior resident, fellows often do not know the learners they are interacting with, which makes learner assessment challenging. In addition, time available for teaching during consultation is generally quite short, and, combined with the sometimes subspecialized nature of the material, engaging in teaching can be a challenge for fellows.

Ultimately, we would argue that many of the factors described as interpersonal factors may fall under the realm of systems issues, and that all these factors are intimately interrelated. For example, when a very busy fellow early in the academic year receives a consult request from an intern without a well-phrased consult question, the intern may perceive some pushback on the part of the fellow and may then choose not to engage the fellow in a teaching interaction when the fellow relays a recommendation. This interaction, rather than fostering positive familiarity may engender some tension, which can extend to future consult interactions. This interrelatedness also represents a major opportunity for improvement, because interventions that reduce a barrier described above can have significant impact by positively affecting multiple aspects of the interaction.

FACTORS AND INTERVENTIONS ENHANCING CONSULTATION

Improving consultation can have a wide array of meanings. Improving the interaction between the fellow and primary team, enhancing the compliance with the consultant's recommendations, increasing teaching and learning, or improving the satisfaction of the patient and care team members all serve to enhance the consult interaction.

Compliance with Consultant Recommendations

To enhance compliance with recommendations, determining what question is being asked is a critical first step. A study by Goldman and colleagues[5] showed that, in 15% of cases, the requesting and consulting physician actually have different senses of the question being asked. Another study looked at factors that increased compliance with the consultant's recommendations and showed that referring physicians comply with the consultant's recommendations between 54% and 95% of the time.[24] Compliance may increase when such consultations are performed the same day or within 24 hours, definitive language is used in recommendations, recommendations are prioritized, and are limited to no more than 5 separate recommendations. In addition, they note that certain clinical factors, such as specifying medication details, for example, dosage, route, frequency, and duration, direct verbal contact, and giving therapeutic as opposed to only diagnostic recommendations, all help to improve compliance.[24]

Communicating Consult Requests

Several approaches focusing on a structured communication of the consult request have been shown to enhance the consultation process (**Table 1**).[15,25–28]

The 5Cs and CONSULT models have focused primarily on communicating the clinical information; our group's approach and the PIQUED framework also focus on enhancing teaching around consultation. 5 Cs is currently the most extensively studied consult communication technique.[22,23] This framework entails providing an introduction, giving a concise clinical story, highlighting the reason and time expected frame for consultation, fostering an open and dynamic conversation, and closing the loop to ensure that all parties understand the next steps. Several studies have shown its benefit, including one assessing intern self-reported preparedness to request consultations and measured communication skills.[23] A total of 96% of interns reported feeling better prepared, and more consultants described interns as better prepared, to request consultations (54% after the intervention versus 27% before).[27]

Our group developed and evaluated a 4-step intervention. First, the supervising resident assisted the intern with identifying a consult question to facilitate reflection in action. Second, the interns were asked to express an interest in learning from the fellow during the consult request. Third, interns were encouraged to engage fellows in teaching, and, fourth, they were asked to bring back a teaching point to rounds to further promote learning. The intervention led to improvement in in-person communication and resident-fellow teaching interactions.[15]

Table 1 Frameworks for calling consultation	
Framework	**Components**
5 Cs[26,27]	• Contact: introduction between consultant and consulting physicians • Communicate: give a concise story and ask focused questions • Core question: specific question with a reasonable timeframe • Collaboration: discussion with changes in diagnostics or management • Closing the loop: ensure both parties are on the same page
PIQUED[28]	• *Prepare*: review necessary information for calling the consult • *Identify*: identify involved parties (patient, trainee, attending physician, consultant) • *Question*: ask focused question • *Urgency*: clarify urgency • *Educational modifications*: let consultant know about your experience or lack thereof, and ask questions that invite teaching • *Debrief*: elicit and provide feedback on the case
CONSULT[25]	• Contact courteously: introduce yourself and team • Orient: provide patient's name, MRN, and location • Narrow question: pose a focused question about diagnosis or treatment • Story: provide a succinct story including pertinent history of present illness, hospital course, and work-up • Urgency: specify whether emergent, very urgent, urgent, or routine • Later: make a follow-up plan and provide contact information • Thank you: show appreciation
MGH framework[15]	• Step 1: Supervising resident assists the intern in coming up with a specific consult question • Step 2: Interns are encouraged to invite teaching during initial consultation • Step 3: Interns are encouraged to ask questions about the case to facilitate teaching when discussing recommendations with fellow • Step 4: Interns share a teaching point they learned from the fellow on rounds

Notably, fellow-directed interventions around receiving consult requests and reducing pushback have not been studied. From our experience we believe that fellows can focus on 4 elements that can enhance the primary team-fellow interaction during the consult request.[8] First, being kind and stating a willingness to help as early as possible during the conversation is a critical step, which helps to transition the conversation from one of negotiation, to a more collaborative process. Second, limiting pushback is important, recognizing that the team requesting a consult is calling for help, even if they are unable to communicate a clear and concise question. Third, avoid asking questions about what can easily be looked up in the medical record. Fourth, set an expectation for an in-person teaching interaction. This last step can help break down barriers to residents engaging fellows in teaching and set positive expectations.

What can program leaders do to enhance communication around consultation in their institutions? In addition to teaching trainees about effective consult communication using the above-mentioned techniques, enhancing familiarity between interns, residents, hospitalists, and fellows can facilitate improved in-person communication. Programs can also focus on familiarizing fellows with primary team structure to allow them better understanding of and access to the teams.

Fellow Teaching Skills

Most fellows are interested in teaching, although many of the barriers described above can pose significant obstacles. A needs assessment of medicine subspecialty fellows revealed that 79% anticipate teaching to be a part of their careers. However, 67% reported that they had received no training focused on teaching skills during their fellowship.[7] Because the subspecialty fellow is often the main consultant interacting with the primary teams on a daily basis, it is critical to develop mechanisms to help fellows grow not only as excellent consultants and physicians but also as educators. To address this opportunity gap, multiple programs aimed at developing fellow teaching skills have been described.[29–33] In addition, as more fellows pursue academic careers as educators, fellowship programs have begun to establish medical education tracks.[34]

Because teaching during inpatient consultation presents unique challenges described above, our group has focused specifically on enhancing fellow teaching skills in this setting. We developed the Fellow as Clinical Teacher (FACT) curriculum, using the PARTNER framework (available for use from MedEdPORTAL) **(Table 2)**.[33,35,36] The curriculum focuses on helping fellows overcome barriers to teaching during consultation. The PARTNER framework helps fellows engage the primary team in active learning in a time-efficient manner. Several studies have evaluated the efficacy of the FACT curriculum demonstrating an improvement in fellow teaching

Table 2
PARTNER framework for teaching during consultation

Components	Examples and Comments
Partner with resident: discuss expectations for learner	"I saw Mr. S and have some thoughts and recommendations but would like to discuss the case with you and do some teaching. Do you have 3 minutes to chat?"
Assess the learner: determine what the learner knows about the case thus far	"What does your team think is going on?"; "How would you interpret the ANA in this setting?"; "How would you distinguish between X and Y in this case?"
Reinforce positives: reinforce positives to create an optimal learning environment	"That's great that you suspected a gout flare, and it sounds like you are very familiar with prednisone, NSAIDs and colchicine for the treatments for gout."
Teaching objectives: identify several teaching points	The learner's knowledge gaps should be assessed with the teaching objectives in mind.
New knowledge: teach general concepts and focus on gaps in learner's understanding	Teaching points to fill in knowledge gaps and correct assumptions should be made concisely, based on learner assessment. Teach and emphasize general concepts when possible. Time should not be spent on what the learner already knows.
Execute recommendations: review consult team's recommendations	Even if discussed in the context of teaching, recommendations should be summarized at the end.
Review: provide time for learner's questions	

Data from Chen DC, Miloslavsky EM, Winn AS, et al. Fellow as Clinical Teacher (FACT) curriculum: improving fellows' teaching skills during inpatient consultation. MedEdPortal 2018;14:10728.

skills as measured by the Objective Structured Teaching Exercise, in which fellows are observed teaching standardized learners.[32,37] Fellows also reported more confidence in their teaching skills and rated the curriculum highly.[33,36] At our institution, the FACT curriculum has been a required part of fellowship curricula in most divisions, and has been well received.

Feedback is critically important to enhance fellow teaching skills. Notably, the ACGME Program Requirements for Graduate Medical Education in Rheumatology state that the program must use performance data to assess the fellow in their teaching skills involving peers and patients.[9] However, there are no recommendations or requirements to provide feedback for improving fellows' teaching skills. Although attendings may oversee fellows giving teaching and instructions to patients, fellows report that direct observation and feedback on their teaching skills is relatively infrequent during fellowship training.[7] In addition, fellows rarely receive feedback from primary teams. This may in part be as a result of the logistical challenges inherent in a large number of residents and hospitalists evaluating a similarly large number of subspecialty fellows. At our institution we have developed and implemented an annual evaluation of medicine subspecialty consult services by hospitalists and housestaff.[34] Responders also have the opportunity to provide feedback to specific fellows. The results are distributed to fellowship program directors with their service identified and all other services de-identified so that comparisons may be made. Fellowship program directors have found this evaluation to be valuable and most have implemented changes in their fellowships based on the results of this evaluation.[38]

Future Directions

Research focusing on inpatient consultation is in its early stages. Over the next decade studies evaluating and categorizing the use of inpatient consultation as well as the extent of teaching on the inpatient services will be helpful. Determining how to test interventions and deciding what outcomes are most useful to measure will be vital moving forward. Should the outcomes be related to the amount of teaching alone, resident and primary team satisfaction, or to the consultant's impression of the interaction? Whether any of these interventions have an impact on patient care outcomes would be important to measure, although demonstrating this effect could be challenging.

Elucidating the relationship between the barriers to teaching and quantifying their effect is critical. For example, illuminating the links between workload, burnout, pushback, perceptions, teaching, and learning will play an important role in identifying and designing effective interventions. In addition, further studies looking into alternative methods of consultations, or different types of workflow, could help enhance the fellow's consult experience. Interventions such as using nurse practitioners and physician assistants has become a growing area of interest across the country. The role of these providers would likely differ based on the specialty and program but could help to augment the fellowship experience. In addition, electronic consultations are used by some health care systems in the outpatient setting as a way to provide brief consultation advice without seeing the patient in person.[39] They are often used either for initial advice or for simple patient consult questions. The possibility of using electronic consults in the inpatient setting to determine whether they could decrease the number of in-person consultations would also be of interest.

The authors believe that a comprehensive approach will likely be required to lead a cultural evolution surrounding the entire process of consultation. Such an approach should include multiple interventions discussed above, including educating primary teams regarding appropriate consult requests and communication, endowing fellows with strategies to overcome barriers faced in the hospital environment, enhancing their teaching skills, augmenting feedback that fellows receive, and considering effective ways of controlling fellow workload. Interventions should be rigorously assessed with multiple outcome measures including primary team and fellow satisfaction, measures of wellness, instruments measuring behavior change and clinical outcomes.

SUMMARY

Inpatient consultation is an increasingly used resource and an important opportunity for teaching and learning. Multiple barriers to fellow teaching and primary team learning during consultation exist in academic medical centers; however, interventions have been shown to reduce these barriers. Such interventions include addressing fellow workload and burnout, enhancing primary team and fellow communication as well as fellow teaching skills. Further research to elucidate the effect of workload and other barriers on the primary team—consultant interaction and testing the effect of comprehensive interventions using robust outcome measures—have the potential to significantly enhance the educational value of consultation.

REFERENCES

1. Stevens J, Nyweide D, Maresh S, et al. Variation in inpatient consultation among older adults in the United States. J Gen Intern Med 2015;30(7):992–9.
2. Adams T, Bonsall J, Hunt D, et al. Hospitalist perspective of interactions with medicine subspecialty consult services. J Hosp Med 2018;13:318–23.
3. Ta K, Gardner G. Evaluation of the activity of an academic rheumatology consult service over 10 years: using data to shape curriculum. J Rheumatol 2007;34(3): 563–6.
4. Cai W, Bruno C, Hagedorn C, et al. Temporal trends over ten years in formal inpatient gastroenterology consultations at an inner city hospital. J Clin Gastroenterol 2003;36:34–8.
5. Goldman L, Lee T, Rudd P. Ten commandments for effective consultations. Arch Intern Med 1983;143(9):1753–5. Available at: http://www.ncbi.nlm.nih.gov/pubmed/6615097. Accessed July 6, 2015.
6. Salerno S, Hurst F, Halvorson S, et al. Principles of effective consultation: an update for the 21st-century consultant. Arch Intern Med 2007;167:271–5.
7. McSparron J, Huang G, Miloslavsky E. Developing internal medicine subspecialty fellows' teaching skills: a needs assessment. BMC Med Educ 2018;18: 221–6.
8. Miloslavsky E, McSparron J, Richards J, et al. Teaching during consultation: factors affecting the resident-fellow teaching interaction. Med Educ 2015;49:717–30.
9. ACGME Program Requirements for Graduate Medical Education in Rheumatology (Internal Medicine). 2017.
10. Howell M. Are you complicating your consults? CRICO.
11. Kolasinski S, Bass A, Kane-Wanger G, et al. Subspecialty choice: why did you become a rheumatologist? Arthritis Rheum 2007;67(8):1546–51.
12. Horn L, Tzanetos K, Thorpe K, et al. Factors associated with the subspecialty choices of internal medicine residents in Canada. BMC Med Educ 2008;8:37.
13. Battafarano D, Ditmyer M, Bolster M, et al. 2015 American College of Rheumatology Workforce Study: supply and demand projections of adult rheumatology workforce, 2015–2030. Arthritis Care Res 2018;70(4):617–26.
14. Miloslavsky E, Puig A. The teaching interaction between internal medicine residents and fellows on the wards: a resident perspective. MedEdPublish; 2014.

15. Gupta S, Alladina J, Heaton K, et al. A randomized trial of an intervention to improve resident-fellow teaching interactions on the wards. BMC Med Educ 2016;16:276–83.
16. Artemeva N, Rachul C, O'Brien B, et al. Situated learning in medical education. Acad Med 2017;92(1):134.
17. Dyrbye L, West C, Satele D, et al. Burnout among U.S. medical students, residents, and early career physicians relative to the general U.S. population. Acad Med 2014;89:443–51.
18. Cubero D, Rego Lins Fumis R, Herick de Sa T, et al. Burnout in medical oncology fellows: a prospective multicenter cohort study in Brazilian institutions. J Cancer Educ 2016;31:582–7.
19. Lally J, Cantillon P. Uncertainty and ambiguity and their association with psychological distress in medical students. Acad Psychiatry 2014;38(3):339–44.
20. Domen RE. The ethics of ambiguity. Acad Pathol 2016;3. 237428951665471.
21. Chan T, Sabir K, Sanhan S, et al. Understanding the impact of residents' interpersonal relationships during emergency department referrals and consultations. J Grad Med Educ 2013;5:576–81.
22. Cruess RL, Cruess SR, Steinert Y. Amending Miller's pyramid to include professional identity formation. Acad Med 2016;91(2):180–5.
23. Miloslavsky EM, Boyer D, Winn AS, et al. Fellows as teachers: raising the educational bar. Ann Am Thorac Soc 2016;13(4):465–8.
24. Cohn S. The role of the medical consultant. Med Clin North Am 2003;87:1–6.
25. Podolsky A, Stern D. The courteous consult: a CONSULT card and training to improve resident consults. J Grad Med Educ 2015;7(1):113–7.
26. Kessler C, Afshar Y, Sardar G, et al. A prospective, randomized, controlled study demonstrating a novel, effective model of transfer of care between physicians: the 5 Cs of consultation. Acad Emerg Med 2012;19(8):968–74.
27. Martin S, Carter K, Hellermann N, et al. The consultation observed simulated clinical experience: training, assessment, and feedback for incoming interns on requesting consultations. Acad Med 2018;93:1814–20.
28. Chan T, Orlich D, Kulasegaram K, et al. Understanding communication between emergency and consulting physicians: a qualitative study that describes and defines the essential elements of the emergency department consultation-referral process for the junior learner. CJEM 2013;15(1):42–51.
29. Kempainen R, Hallstrand T, Culver B, et al. Fellows as teachers: the teacher-assistant experience during pulmonary subspecialty training. Chest 2005;128:401–6.
30. Rosenbaum M, Rowat J, Ferguson K, et al. Developing future faculty: a program targeting internal medicine fellows' teaching skills. J Grad Med Educ 2011;3:302–8.
31. Backes C, Reber K, Trittmann J, et al. Fellows as teachers: a model to enhance pediatric resident education. Med Educ Online 2011;16. https://doi.org/10.3402/meo.v16i0.7205.
32. Tofil N, Peterson D, Harrington K, et al. A novel iterative-learner simulation model: fellows as teachers. J Grad Med Educ 2014;6:127–32.
33. Rivera V, Yukawa M, Aronson L, et al. Teaching geriatric fellows how to teach: a needs assessment targeting geriatrics fellowship program directors. J Am Geriatr Soc 2014;62:2377–82.
34. Adamson R, Goodman R, Kritek P, et al. Training the teachers. The clinician-educator track of the University of Washington Pulmonary and Critical Care Medicine Fellowship Program. Ann Am Thorac Soc 2015;12(4):480–5.

35. Chen D, Miloslavsky E, Winn A, et al. Fellow as Clinical Teacher (FACT) curriculum: improving fellows' teaching skills during inpatient consultation. MedEdPORTAL 2018;14:10728.
36. Miloslavsky E, Degnan K, McNeill J, et al. Use of Fellow as Clinical Teacher (FACT) curriculum for teaching during consultation: effect on subspecialty fellow teaching skills. J Grad Med Educ 2017;9:345–50.
37. Miloslavsky E, Criscione-Schreiber L, Jonas B, et al. Fellow as teacher curriculum: improving rheumatology fellows' teaching skills during inpatient consultation. Arthritis Care Res 2016;68(6):877–81.
38. Miloslavsky E, Chang Y. Development and evaluation of a novel survey tool assessing inpatient consult service performance. J Grad Med Educ 2017;9(6): 759–62.
39. Wrenn K, Catschegn S, Cruz M, et al. Analysis of an electronic consultation program at an academic medical centre: primary care provider questions, specialist responses, and primary care provider actions. J Telemed Telecare 2017;23(2): 217–24.

Learning to Critically Appraise Rheumatic Disease Literature
Educational Opportunities During Training and into Practice

Juliet Aizer, MD, MPH[a],*, Julie A. Schell, EdD, MS, BS[b,c], Marianna B. Frey, BA[d], Michael D. Tiongson, BA[e], Lisa A. Mandl, MD, MPH[a]

KEYWORDS

- Medical education (graduate medical education, continuing medical education)
- Critical appraisal • Epidemiology • Biostatistics • Retrieval practice
- Self-determination theory • Communities of practice

KEY POINTS

- Equipping and motivating clinicians to critically appraise the literature supports optimal patient care.
- Conceptual frameworks of Retrieval Enhanced Learning, Self-Determination Theory, and Communities of Practice can inform design of educational approaches to promote critical appraisal in practice.
- HSS CLASS-Rheum® is a learning tool that can be used to help rheumatologists learn skills for critical appraisal through retrieval practice.
- Combining retrieval practice with opportunities for connection through Peer Instruction, journal clubs, and other forums can support engagement and internalization of motivation, promoting persistence with critical appraisal in practice.

[a] Rheumatology, Weill Cornell Medicine, Hospital for Special Surgery, 535 East 70th Street, New York, NY 10021, USA; [b] School of Design and Creative Technologies, College of Education, Dual Appointment, The University of Texas at Austin, Office of Strategy and Policy, 405 West 25th Street, Stop F0900, Austin, TX 78705, USA; [c] Associate with Mazur Group, John A. Paulson School of Engineering and Applied Sciences, Harvard University, Cambridge, MA, USA; [d] Rheumatology, Hospital for Special Surgery, 535 East 70th Street, New York, NY 10021, USA; [e] Albany Medical College, 43 New Scotland Avenue, Albany, NY 12208, USA
* Corresponding author.
E-mail address: aizerj@hss.edu

Rheum Dis Clin N Am 46 (2020) 85–102
https://doi.org/10.1016/j.rdc.2019.09.006
0889-857X/20/© 2019 Elsevier Inc. All rights reserved.

Video content accompanies this article at http://www.rheumatic.theclinics. com.

THE NEED FOR CRITICAL APPRAISAL EDUCATION

There have been tremendous scientific advances in rheumatology over the past decades. New diagnostic tools and therapeutic approaches have been developed, allowing us to prognosticate, communicate with, and treat patients better than ever. For patients to benefit from these advances, physicians cannot rely solely on their medical school and postgraduate training; it is imperative that physicians continue to learn.[1] With the advent of online publications, there has been an explosion in the volume of literature, making it more important to be able to identify which are the valid, high-quality studies.[2] Despite this, negative studies remain less likely to be published[3,4]; recognizing this type of publication bias as well as the limitations and potential biases of available data must be considered.[5] Rheumatologists must parse the literature and choose which data to act on. For example, it is crucial to identify high-quality studies to best determine which biologic would be most effective for a specific patient with nonradiographic spondyloarthritis,[6] or to evaluate the generalizability of published data when deciding whether a patient with gout and a history of ischemic chest pain should be given febuxostat.[7] Rheumatologists designing research or serving in administrative roles that influence clinical guidelines and policies should apply critical appraisal as well. Although literature reviews can be key resources for answering questions in lieu of reviewing primary data, selective assembly, bias, lack of applicability, and/or absence of the most current data may present significant drawbacks. Clinicians must be adept at identifying appropriate sources, properly interpreting evidence, and accurately sharing information with patients to optimize care in an information-saturated age.

Recognizing that all rheumatologists need to answer patient-centered questions, the Accreditation Council for Graduate Medical Education (ACGME) considers the ability to critique specialized scientific literature effectively to be a key characteristic of rheumatology trainees who are ready for unsupervised practice.[8]

Critical appraisal, the "…application of rules of evidence … to assess the validity of the data, completeness of reporting, methods and procedures, conclusions, compliance with ethical standards, etc.,"[9] requires a specific set of knowledge and skills that can feel inaccessible to many physicians. If one is not fluent in the vocabulary of epidemiology and biostatistics, it can be bewildering to try to interpret, critique, and apply information from the literature. It takes time and resources to acquire the knowledge and skills required to critically appraise the literature, and additional time to maintain them.

Equipping rheumatologists with critical appraisal knowledge and skills will improve patient care only if critical appraisal is applied in clinical practice. Time constraints, insufficient support, false beliefs about evidence-based medicine, and limited critical appraisal skills have been identified as the most common barriers to health care providers' performance of evidence-based practice.[10,11] It is therefore crucial to integrate critical appraisal skills into a framework that supports their implementation.

THE NEED FOR RESOURCES FOR CRITICAL APPRAISAL EDUCATION IN RHEUMATOLOGY TRAINING PROGRAMS

Critical appraisal education at the undergraduate and graduate training levels is incompletely described in the literature. Available evidence indicates this topic is generally included in these curricula, but there is a large degree of variability in how, when, and where critical appraisal is taught.[12–15] Basic epidemiology and biostatistics are included on US Medical Licensing Examinations,[16] but the small number of questions on these topics means it is possible to pass these examinations without correctly answering these questions. Despite inclusion of critical appraisal topics in undergraduate medical education curricula and residency training programs, trainees often demonstrate limited critical appraisal skills at the start of their rheumatology training. Thus, training programs should be structured to designate time and direct trainees to build critical appraisal skills, but it has been unclear how these skills should be taught.

Journal clubs involving use of critical appraisal are common components of training programs, but outcome data on their effects on subsequent evidence-based practice are limited.[17] To improve the impact of journal clubs on evidence-based practice, Alguire[17] suggested incorporating and formally evaluating adult learning principles in trainee journal clubs. A Cochrane systematic review found that, although teaching critical appraisal to medical professionals may improve knowledge, there was a lack of high-quality studies evaluating changes in process of care or patient outcomes after critical appraisal teaching.[18] The investigators recognized a need for rigorous randomized trials of educational programs for critical appraisal informed by appropriate learning theories.

Educational resources available through the American College of Rheumatology (ACR) support trainees' achievement of core competencies and specific skills such as ultrasound, bone densitometry, and practice management.[1] Resources for helping trainees learn elements of critical appraisal, however, are lacking. The ACR/Association of Rheumatology Health Professionals Annual Scientific Meeting[19] includes a few sessions about statistical approaches, but these are generally targeted at researchers. Guided poster tours direct attendees' attention to high-impact data but are not intended to teach critical appraisal. The ACR Continuing Assessment Review and Evaluation (CARE) modules include a few questions on epidemiology and biostatistics each year, but this handful of questions are necessarily narrow in scope.

The ACR has acknowledged the lack of curricular resources dedicated to critical appraisal in rheumatology training programs and the importance of addressing it. To fill this resource gap, the ACR recently embarked on a new initiative called Rheum4Science, to provide Web-based modules on elements of basic and clinical science that will allow asynchronous learning with interactive elements.[20] Some Rheum4Science modules will help promote critical appraisal, as there is overlap in the knowledge and skills relevant to both performing clinical research and critically appraising research publications.

RETRIEVAL ENHANCED LEARNING, SELF-DETERMINATION THEORY, AND COMMUNITIES OF PRACTICE AS FRAMEWORKS FOR EDUCATIONAL APPROACHES TO CRITICAL APPRAISAL

Conceptual frameworks in education can serve as helpful lenses through which to view a problem and then design educational solutions.[21,22] In considering the challenges to teaching and learning critical appraisal, conceptual frameworks of Retrieval Enhanced Learning, Self-Determination Theory (Motivation), and Communities of Practice can guide effective interventions (**Fig. 1**).

Retrieval Enhanced Learning (Retrieval Practice)

Educational research demonstrates that learning approaches that require active learning, encoding, processing, and retrieval of learning lead to stronger memory, long-term retention, construction of new knowledge, and the ability to flexibly use

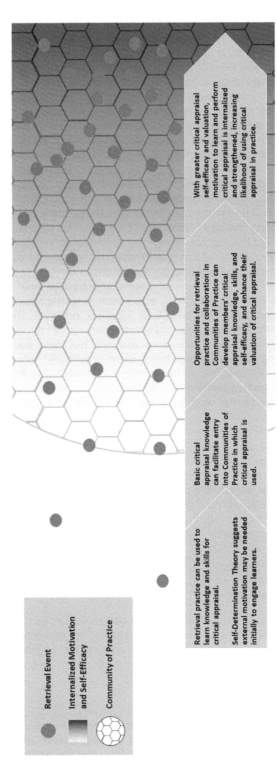

Fig. 1. Model of the integration of Retrieval Enhanced Learning Theory (Retrieval Practice), Self-Determination Theory (Motivation), and Communities of Practice to promote learning and application of critical appraisal.

that knowledge in new and unfamiliar contexts.[23–28] This is in contrast to more prevalent but less effective transmissionist approaches to education that rely on experts "transmitting" knowledge to passive learners.[29]

Empirical evidence has established that testing does not simply measure knowledge, it changes the memory of the test taker, thereby causing learning.[23] Recalling information from memory, referred to as "retrieval practice," promotes deep learning, and can do so more effectively than reading, reviewing, and re-reading materials. Retrieval practice has been proven to promote long-term retention of content across a range of complexity.[26,30] Beyond simply improving recall of an item, retrieval practice also promotes further encoding and processing of information and subsequent transfer of learning to different contexts,[28] allowing the knowledge gained through testing to be used flexibly in future situations with new and unfamiliar material (eg, knowledge about echolocation in bats can be transferred and applied to sonar in submarines).[23] Recalling knowledge in one domain can facilitate recall of proximate or related knowledge, even if it is not part of the tested item.[31]

There are hundreds of ways to engage learners in retrieval practice. Multiple-choice questions and short-answer formats can both be effective.[26] One approach involves posing a question, allowing time for the learner to recall and formulate an answer, and then providing feedback on the correct answer. When accompanied by feedback, retrieval supports and strengthens subsequent storage in memory. Feedback is important because it allows the learner to correct any errors and confidently maintain correct responses. Effective feedback includes correct answer identification and explanatory feedback for why that answer is correct. Explanatory feedback is particularly important for transfer of learning to new contexts.[32] The structure of the retrieval practice can enhance learning; including repetition of the question, providing time between repeated retrieval attempts (spacing), and varying the type of retrieval activities can enhance the effects.[33] When the structure includes retrieval with feedback, learners are better able to engage in self-appraisal, self-monitoring, and self-regulation of learning.[33,34] Such metacognitive abilities are linked to a range of benefits, including deeper problem-solving skills and the ability to apply and use that learning more effectively in future situations.

This understanding of how tests can promote learning can inform the design of educational formats to improve retention and subsequent transfer of critical appraisal knowledge and skills.

Self-Determination Theory (Motivation)

Considering how to effectively motivate learners to engage in development of critical appraisal skills (through retrieval practice or otherwise) and use critical appraisal in practice is key when designing educational interventions. Deci and Ryan's Self-Determination Theory provides a helpful framework to do so.[35–38]

In some circumstances, learner motivation is driven by the appeal of the activity itself, rather than by a consequence of the activity. This "intrinsic motivation" can be quite powerful; when possible, educational tasks should be designed to maximize intrinsic appeal. Perceived competence (self-efficacy, the belief one can perform a task successfully)[39,40] and autonomy (self-direction, choice) have been demonstrated to be powerful internal motivators. Instilling a sense of self-efficacy for critical appraisal, and recognition of the ability to direct one's own learning through critical appraisal, have the potential to motivate use of critical appraisal in practice.

Because of required roles and responsibilities, most adults' activities are not primarily intrinsically motivated. Self-Determination Theory categorizes all forms of motivation that are not strictly intrinsic as forms of "extrinsic motivation." The extent to which extrinsic motivations are self-determined, or internalized, has significant range. At one end of the continuum, behaviors are performed to satisfy an external demand, whereas at the other end of the continuum, behaviors are performed voluntarily, to obtain an outcome one personally values. Internalization of values is associated with enhanced engagement, persistence, and sense of well-being. Supporting senses of relatedness (belonging or connectedness), competence, and autonomy can foster internalization of values; we see that people are more motivated to perform a behavior when

1. they sense that behavior is valued by others they want to feel connected to
2. they sense they possess the relevant skills to perform it successfully
3. they personally appreciate the worth of the behavior

This framework can inform design of educational programs to enhance interest in, valuing of, and self-efficacy for critical appraisal, thereby promoting use of critical appraisal in practice. One may first be exposed to an activity in response to an external prompt, but then appreciate it as intrinsically interesting or personally valuable, leading to internalization of the motivation.

Communities of Practice

The establishment of "Communities of Practice" can help cultivate learning of critical appraisal skills in current and future generations of rheumatologists and advance the use of critical appraisal in rheumatology.

Emphasizing the social and situated nature of learning, Lave and Wenger[41] described the educational framework of Communities of Practice as groups of people who "share and develop an overlapping knowledge base, set of beliefs, values, history and experiences focused on a common practice and/or mutual enterprise".[42] Communities of Practice are defined by 3 key features:

1. a shared domain of knowledge
2. a community of individuals working within the domain
3. the development of tools, resources, and innovations that advance the domain

Individuals interested in joining a Community of Practice move from peripheral participation as novice members, toward full membership as they acquire knowledge, skills, and a sense of shared identity or membership with the group. An individual's learning can be seen as a journey through a landscape of Communities of Practice, modulated by the individual's interest and access.

Communities of Practice can be problematic, as they can be exclusionary; there can be barriers to access and historical power relationships can be reinforced.[43] There can be a sense of discomfort when one is at the margins of a Community of Practice, unsure of the rules and unfamiliar with the language.[22,44,45] Sustaining a productive Community of Practice is dependent on new generations of members joining. "Participation, or coparticipation, with fellow learners and more senior members of the community...deepens the sense of engagement."[42]

Learning and applying critical appraisal can be seen as occurring within Communities of Practice; the domain is critical appraisal, the community is the network of individuals who engage in critical appraisal together, and the practice is the curation, development, and use of tools and resources to help advance critical appraisal. Communities of Practice can provide an infrastructure for learning, instilling a sense of the value and supporting the development of critical appraisal. As critical appraisal knowledge, skills, and values, are acquired, rheumatologists can move toward full membership in these Communities. An important educational goal is to actively assist novice learners to join these Communities.

DESIGNING CURRICULAR SUPPORT FOR CRITICAL APPRAISAL DURING TRAINING: HOSPITAL FOR SPECIAL SURGERY CRITICAL LITERATURE ASSESSMENT SKILLS SUPPORT-RHEUMATOLOGY (HSS CLASS-RHEUM®)

Application of the educational frameworks of Retrieval Enhanced Learning, Self-Determination Theory, and Communities of Practice can be seen in the design and implementation of a new learning tool called Hospital for Special Surgery Critical Literature Assessment Skills Support–Rheumatology (HSS CLASS-Rheum).

Identification of Learning Objectives

To establish which study designs are particularly pertinent to rheumatologists, our group reviewed 30% of the clinical research articles (excluding opinion pieces, letters, and reviews) published in *Annals of Rheumatic Disease, Arthritis and Rheumatology*, and *Arthritis Care and Research* over a 9-month period. We selected these journals based on impact factor, their focus on original research, and broad coverage of general rheumatology.[46] Registries, cohorts, and case control studies were most prevalent, followed by systematic reviews and meta-analyses, case series, and randomized controlled trials (RCTs) (**Fig. 2**). Although RCTs are generally thought of as providing a higher level of evidence, the high frequency of cohorts and case control studies in the rheumatic disease literature indicates that rheumatologists in particular must have a thorough understanding of these study designs. We used this information to inform the development of a set of key learning

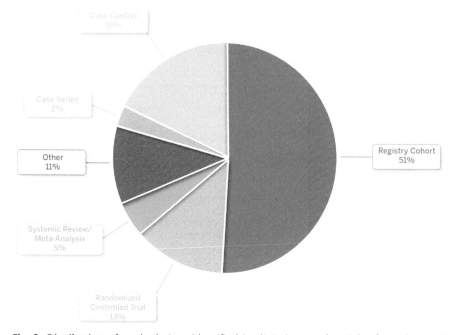

Fig. 2. Distribution of study designs identified in clinical research articles from rheumatic disease literature.

objectives reflecting these specific needs, to prepare rheumatology trainees to critically appraise the clinical rheumatic disease literature.

Application of Retrieval Enhanced Learning (Retrieval Practice)

Given the proven benefits of retrieval practice, we developed a question-based curricular tool using varied response types. Recognizing the diversity of programs in terms of availability and expertise of faculty, and the different ways trainees' time is organized, we designed HSS CLASS-Rheum to optimize flexibility in implementation. We used a Web-based assessment system capable of supporting retrieval practice through various question types and modes of delivery. HSS CLASS-Rheum can be deployed in 3 ways:

1. Individual, Asynchronous
2. Individual, Synchronous
3. Team-based with Peer Instruction (**Box 1**)

We constructed introductory materials in print and video format (Video 1), explaining the purpose and use of HSS CLASS-Rheum.

The HSS CLASS-Rheum questions are grouped in 2 Question Sets, each composed of 10 thematic modules, with 3 to 9 American Board of Internal Medicine/National Board of Medical Examiners (ABIM/NBME)-style[47] multiple choice or numeric short-answer questions per module (**Box 2**). The 2 Question Sets mirror each other, being composed of different questions addressing the same learning objectives ("isomorphic questions"). Use of isomorphic questions enhances learning by providing another retrieval opportunity in a new context.

When using HSS CLASS-Rheum, each trainee is instructed to read the question, consider their answer, and enter a response. HSS CLASS-Rheum provides immediate feedback to the trainee on whether the submitted answer is correct, explanatory feedback through an answer rationale stating what the correct answer is and why, and information about why the distractors are incorrect. Immediate feedback has been shown to improve recall, and is especially important for multiple-choice questions

---

Box 1
Hospital for Special Surgery Critical Literature Assessment Skills Support–Rheumatology (HSS CLASS-Rheum) modes for use

Individual, Asynchronous
- Trainees individually complete HSS CLASS-Rheum modules on their own time
- Provides trainees with the most flexibility in choosing when to complete modules

Individual, Synchronous
- Trainees individually complete HSS CLASS-Rheum modules during a set time, generally when they are scheduled to meet together
- Can be followed by group discussion to further support learning
- Provides trainees with dedicated time to complete modules

Team-Based, with Peer Instruction
- Trainees are grouped into teams and go through 2 rounds of questioning
- First they answer the module individually, without peer input
- Then trainees discuss the questions with their teammates and submit a team answer for each question
- Provides fellows with an opportunity to engage in Peer Instruction, associated with increases in problem-solving skills, conceptual knowledge of complex subjects, and performance on standardized assessments

> **Box 2**
> **HSS CLASS-Rheum modules**
>
> • Data and Distributions
>
> • Case Series
>
> • Cohort Studies
>
> • Case Control Studies
>
> • Randomized Controlled Trials
>
> • Crossover Studies
>
> • Non-Inferiority Trials
>
> • Survival Analysis
>
> • Test Characteristics and Instrument Performance
>
> • Systematic Reviews and Meta-Analyses
>
> Each of the 2 Question Sets is organized into these 10 modules. The 2 Question Sets address the same learning objectives with isomorphic questions.

that can otherwise lead to learning incorrect information.[23] This feedback can stimulate the trainee to reflect on their understanding, identify knowledge gaps or misunderstandings, and address them.

Application of Self-Determination Theory

Program directors are able to modulate external motivation for their trainees' completion of HSS CLASS-Rheum questions; it can be deemed a training program requirement (which would more strongly drive completion of assigned modules) or an optional resource for interested trainees (which may then only be used by trainees who already have sufficiently internalized motivation for learning critical appraisal).

Program directors have access to their trainees' performance in HSS CLASS-Rheum. This allows program directors to recognize their trainees' learning needs and monitor them longitudinally to determine whether these needs have been effectively addressed. Program directors can potentially establish external motivation by requiring trainees to repeat HSS CLASS-Rheum modules or whole Question Sets.

To help trainees appreciate the relevance and application of the content and to promote motivation to engage in the learning, all HSS CLASS-Rheum questions are framed as cases within the scope of rheumatology trainees' experiences. Questions highlight situations in which critical appraisal informs best care for patients with rheumatic disease.

Application of Communities of Practice

HSS CLASS-Rheum can be used in formats and settings that involve and foster collaborative learning and application of critical appraisal in practice, in effect introducing trainees to benefits of critical appraisal Communities of Practice, and potentially helping such Communities to emerge and develop. Use of HSS CLASS-Rheum with Peer Instruction and journal clubs are 2 ways to support development of critical appraisal Communities of Practice using HSS CLASS-Rheum.

Peer Instruction[33,48–51] is a teaching method shown to promote learner engagement, conceptual understanding, and problem-solving skills, particularly in science.[33,52] Peer Instruction offers a way to deliver instruction that is directly aligned with the benefits of retrieval practice, including repeated retrieval attempts, immediate and explanatory feedback, timing and spacing of retrieval, and variable retrieval activities. This method involves a sequence of 7 steps (**Box 3**), including both individual thought and sharing of knowledge and ideas.[52] Empirical evidence has demonstrated that when Peer Instruction is used, learning outcomes improve, including gains in conceptual understanding, academic performance, and positive feelings toward content.[53] The HSS CLASS-Rheum Team format is designed to support Peer Instruction techniques.

Aligning HSS CLASS-Rheum module content with common study designs facilitates their use in conjunction with a journal club. Trainees can read a relevant article from the rheumatic disease literature and complete the HSS CLASS-Rheum module for that study design, either in advance of a small group discussion or at the beginning of a journal club session. Pairing HSS CLASS-Rheum with an article can highlight important methodologies in the article and incorporate additional retrieval of critical appraisal knowledge. Retrieval is first attempted when each individual trainee initially critically appraises the article before discussion. Secondary retrieval attempts occur while answering the HSS CLASS-Rheum questions. A third set of retrieval attempts can be prompted in the journal club discussion. Some examples of questions that can prompt learning through retrieval practice in journal club discussions are provided in **Box 4**.

EXPERIENCE WITH HSS CLASS-RHEUM

HSS CLASS-Rheum was piloted in 6 adult and pediatric rheumatology training programs between January and June 2016.[54] Trainees participating in this pilot demonstrated sustained gains of critical appraisal knowledge and skills after participating in sequential HSS CLASS-Rheum Question Sets. Trainees attained higher mean percentage of answers correct on the second HSS CLASS-Rheum Question Set compared with the first ($P = .04$), with 14% of participants' scores increasing by more than 20 percentage points[54]; 88% of participating trainees reported HSS CLASS-Rheum addressed a gap in their rheumatology training. Participants considered HSS CLASS-Rheum useful or very useful for learning epidemiology and biostatistics. Although other experiences may have also contributed to learning during

---

Box 3
Steps in Peer Instruction

1. Question posed (1 minute)

2. Students given time to think (1 minute)

3. Students record individual answers [optional[a]]

4. Students convince their neighbors—peer instruction (1–2 minutes)

5. Students record revised answers [optional]

6. Feedback to teacher: tally of answers

7. Explanation of correct answer (2+ minutes)

[a] Mazur has emphasized that step 3 promotes learning and therefore should not be skipped.

The process of Peer Instruction has been outlined by Eric Mazur as 7 steps that can optimize learning outcomes.

Data from Mazur E. Peer Instruction: A User's Manual. Upper Saddle River: Prentice Hall, Inc.; 1997.

Box 4
Examples of questions to promote learning through retrieval practice in journal club discussions

- "What is the study design?"
- "Do the participants in this study resemble patients in your clinic?"
- "In what ways could this have biased the study?"
- "How concerned are you that a confounding factor might have affected these results?"
- "What conclusions would you draw from this study?"
- "How might you apply the results of this study in patient care, or in directing future research?"

Targeted questions in journal club discussions can promote further learning through repeated retrieval practice. Example queries from the creators of HSS CLASS-Rheum can be particularly beneficial when used in conjunction with appropriate online modules.

---

the intervening months, these data are consistent with meaningful learning over this interval with effective learning transfer.

Program directors involved in the pilot of HSS CLASS-Rheum also reported that the modules filled an unmet need in their programs, helping them better understand trainees' epidemiology and statistics knowledge, or lack thereof, and providing detailed explanations of pertinent material. In programs that already had courses covering critical appraisal material, program directors praised the modules as a useful complement to solidify knowledge. Some participants suggested future alignment of HSS CLASS-Rheum questions with a structured epidemiology curriculum in which additional content is delivered before completing each HSS CLASS-Rheum module. Publications referenced in the HSS CLASS-Rheum materials or Rheum4Science modules could be used to serve this purpose.

Trainees felt that by framing questions in a rheumatologic context, HSS CLASS-Rheum enhanced their sense of the learning experience's relevance. Trainees also liked using HSS CLASS-Rheum with Peer Instruction in the Team format, and/or in association with journal club discussions. Program directors cited the benefits of setting aside time to meet as a group and work on the modules. They felt these targeted discussions were enjoyable and informative, allowing trainees to clarify and address areas of uncertainty. Participants expressed the hope that future trainees from smaller programs might be able to connect to HSS CLASS-Rheum online in virtual journal clubs coordinated between medical centers. Using HSS CLASS-Rheum in these ways (with Peer Instruction, journal club discussions, or small group discussions of the HSS CLASS-Rheum modules themselves) participants can be seen as working collaboratively in emergent Communities of Practice.

Overall, HSS CLASS-Rheum provides an example of the way in which educational frameworks and validated educational practices could be leveraged to improve rheumatology trainees' grasp and future application of critical appraisal.

THE NEED FOR CRITICAL APPRAISAL EDUCATION AFTER TRAINING

With enhancements to critical appraisal teaching in training, future rheumatologists may enter the workforce with greater knowledge and skills in this area, as well as attitudes that support critical appraisal in practice. However, the current workforce lacks skills needed for critical appraisal.[55–57] This is a major barrier toward teaching critical appraisal skills to the next generation. Local faculty may not be or feel able to teach critical appraisal, and this may telegraph a hidden curriculum to trainees and others in the medical community that critical appraisal skills are not necessary and/or that critical appraisal skills are too difficult to learn.

APPLYING EDUCATIONAL THEORIES TO CRITICAL APPRAISAL EDUCATION AFTER TRAINING

Retrieval Enhanced Learning theory, Self-Determination Theory (Motivation), and Communities of Practice are useful lenses for understanding and designing critical appraisal education during and after training. After training, retrieval practice remains a useful approach to promote encoding and processing of information and subsequent transfer of learning to different contexts. Factors affecting motivation for learning critical appraisal, however, can shift after formal training is complete, and access to Communities of Practice can be different for faculty than for trainees.

Motivating Factors Related to Learning Critical Appraisal After Training

To ensure uptake of critical appraisal skills, physicians must be motivated to learn and maintain them. Institutional requirements, Continuing Medical Education (CME), and/or Maintenance of Certification (MOC) are potential external motivators after training, but as acknowledged by the Accreditation Council for Continuing Medical Education (ACCME), "top-down mandates for education are not only typically ineffective, but create cynicism that erodes clinicians' trust and engagement in their continuing medical education."[58]

Retrieval Practice Opportunities for Learning Critical Appraisal After Training

Recognizing that "professional development is most effective when the clinician is engaging in it for a purpose and when the material is meaningful and relevant to her or his scope of practice; is presented by a trusted authority; engages learners actively; and includes feedback, reflection, and reinforcement,"[59] there has been an effort to tie CME credit to relevant activities. Providing opportunities for self-assessment and retrieval practice, multiple-choice questions are provided in conjunction with some journal articles for MOC and CME credit. Rather than focusing exclusively on direct recall of conclusions stated in the journal article, asking some questions addressing critical appraisal skills and their application to the articles would expand the scope of the educational activity to help physicians raise their awareness of gaps in their critical appraisal knowledge and skills, while emphasizing relevance and bolstering learning.

Communities of Practice for Learning Critical Appraisal After Training

To foster internalization of motivation, Communities of Practice are potentially vital.[60–63] Communities of Practice can encourage adoption of values, and provide opportunities for collaboration. Convening journal clubs on a regular schedule is one way to "develop institutional culture and habits of evidence appraisal,"[64] which can be seen as an example of a Community of Practice. Providing food and time for socializing can potentially increase attendance in these forums.[64] Enhanced social or academic status associated with demonstration of appraisal, particularly high-quality appraisal, are cited as potential positive incentives to participation in appraisal activities.[64]

Access to Communities of Practice can be an issue; creating specific infrastructure is important to facilitate bringing people together into these Communities. Not everyone has a local forum; online technologies can create virtual spaces to expand opportunities for rheumatologists to connect with colleagues to critically appraise the literature and in doing so, develop and reinforce critical appraisal skills in online Communities of Practice.[65] A good example of such a virtual Community of Practice is #RheumJC,[60] an innovative, monthly journal club hosted on Twitter, which has allowed international participation in structured discussions of relevant rheumatology research.[61] Using a mailing list and tweets, cofounders announce the date and time of the next meeting, as well as the paper for discussion, which is often available through open-access for a short time before the meeting.[61] Using their personal twitter accounts, interested individuals can join 1 of 2 live, 1-hour feeds hosted by #RheumJC cofounders, sometimes with invited authors,[55] or post to the feed anytime over a 24-hour open period. As of December 2017, 646 individuals from 36 countries had joined #RheumJC discussions and the #RheumJC Twitter account had more than 2700 followers.[63] These virtual journal clubs have received positive feedback, with more than 85% of respondents reporting that they were satisfied or very satisfied with the discussions, and 37% indicating the information discussed had influenced their clinical practice.[62,63] However, it must also be acknowledged that virtual spaces are less comfortable for some and thus are not the definitive solution for all.

We are optimistic about the potential for a variety of Communities of Practice to instill the value of critical appraisal and promote performance of critical appraisal. External prompts or requirements can provide important exposure. Teaching fundamental critical appraisal knowledge and skills in rheumatology training may help novices over the threshold[44] and into these Communities. Analogously, properly designed CME activities could help practicing rheumatologists join critical appraisal Communities of Practice.

Observing and connecting with others who are performing critical appraisal, developing a sense of personal self-efficacy for critical appraisal, and internalizing its value are all key for use of critical appraisal in practice.

SUMMARY

Rheumatologists must perform critical appraisal to provide optimal patient care. Currently, there is a dearth of validated and effective resources to teach and encourage critical appraisal in rheumatology. Conceptual frameworks of Retrieval Enhanced Learning, Self-Determination Theory, and Communities of Practice can inform design of educational approaches such as HSS CLASS-Rheum to promote development of critical appraisal skills and use of critical appraisal in practice. Engaging trainees and rheumatologists in activities that involve retrieval of critical appraisal knowledge has the potential to increase their learning and ability to use that material in the future. Acquisition of basic critical appraisal knowledge through retrieval practice can facilitate rheumatologists' entry to critical appraisal Communities of Practice. Opportunities for trainees and rheumatologists to connect through Peer Instruction, journal clubs, and a variety of virtual forums can help expand formation of and access to critical appraisal Communities of Practice. Critical appraisal Communities of Practice can foster internalization of motivation for critical appraisal, and ultimately promote application of critical appraisal in patient care.

DISCLOSURES

J. Aizer: Hospital for Special Surgery (employment, salary), Hospital for Special Surgery Academy of Medical Educators (grant support), Weill Cornell Medical College Clinical & Translational Science Center NIH UL1TR000457, Weill Cornell Medicine –

Nanette Laitman Education Scholar in Entrepreneurship (salary support), Rheum4Science (Clinical Science module designer, stipend for module development), American College of Rheumatology – previous chair of the Continuous Professional Development Subcommittee and the CARE Development Group. J. Schell: The University of Texas at Austin (employment, salary), The University of Texas at Austin (clinical faculty, 0%), Harvard University (courtesy appointment, 0%). M. Frey: HSS Academy of Medical Educators (salary). M. Tiongson: HSS Academy of Medical Educators (salary). L. Mandl: Hospital for Special Surgery (employment, salary), Hospital for Special Surgery Academy of Medical Educators (grant support), Weill Cornell Medical College Clinical & Translational Science Center NIH UL1TR000457, Rheum4Science (Clinical Science module designer, stipend for module development), Associate Editor, *Annals of Internal Medicine* (salary), Author, Up-To-Date (royalties).

ACKNOWLEDGMENTS

The authors thank Dr Pascale Schwab, Dr Christopher E. Collins, Dr Karina Torralba, Dr Jessica R. Berman, Dr Anne R. Bass, Dr Lisa Criscione-Schreiber, Dr Carol Mancuso, Dr Michael Pillinger, Dr Alexa Adams, Jackie Szymonifka, Rima Abhyankar, Kelly McHugh, and Dr Nathaniel Hupert for their input on the HSS CLASS-Rheum tool, the rheumatology trainees who have used HSS CLASS-Rheum and provided input, and Dr Stephen A. Paget and the HSS Academy of Medical Educators for supporting the HSS CLASS-Rheum project.

SUPPLEMENTARY DATA

Supplementary data related to this article can be found online at https://doi.org/10.1016/j.rdc.2019.09.006.

REFERENCES

1. Lim SY, Bolster MB. Challenges in optimizing medical education for rheumatologists. Rheum Dis Clin North Am 2019;45(1):127–44.
2. Landhuis E. Scientific literature: information overload. Nature 2016;535(7612):457–8.
3. Ziai H, Zhang R, Chan A-W, et al. Search for unpublished data by systematic reviewers: an audit. BMJ Open 2017;7(10):e017737.
4. Song F, Parekh S, Hooper L, et al. Dissemination and publication of research findings: an updated review of related biases. Health Technol Assess 2010;14(8):iii, ix-xi, 1-193.
5. Every-Palmer S, Howick J. How evidence-based medicine is failing due to biased trials and selective publication: EBM fails due to biased trials and selective publication. J Eval Clin Pract 2014;20(6):908–14.
6. Deodhar A, Gensler LS, Kay J, et al. A 52-week randomized placebo-controlled trial of certolizumab pegol in non-radiographic axial spondyloarthritis. Arthritis Rheumatol 2019. https://doi.org/10.1002/art.40866.
7. White WB, Saag KG, Becker MA, et al. Cardiovascular safety of febuxostat or allopurinol in patients with gout. N Engl J Med 2018;378(13):1200–10.
8. The Accreditation Council for Graduate Medical Education. The American Board of Internal Medicine. The internal medicine subspecialty milestones project 2015. Available at: https://www.acgme.org/Portals/0/PDFs/Milestones/InternalMedicine SubspecialtyMilestones.pdf. Accessed February 27, 2019.
9. Porta MS. A dictionary of epidemiology. In: Sander G, Miguel H, dos Santos Silva I, et al, editors. 4th edition. New York: Oxford University Press; 2001.

Available at: https://www.ncbi.nlm.nih.gov/nlmcatalog/101315961. Accessed March 22, 2019.

10. Hecht L, Buhse S, Meyer G. Effectiveness of training in evidence-based medicine skills for healthcare professionals: a systematic review. BMC Med Educ 2016;16. https://doi.org/10.1186/s12909-016-0616-2.

11. Zwolsman SE, van Dijk N, Waard MW. Barriers to the use of evidence-based medicine: knowledge and skills, attitude, and external factors. Perspect Med Educ 2013;2(1):4–13.

12. Ahmadi S-F, Baradaran HR, Ahmadi E. Effectiveness of teaching evidence-based medicine to undergraduate medical students: a BEME systematic review. Med Teach 2015;37(1):21–30.

13. Maggio LA, Tannery NH, Chen HC, et al. Evidence-based medicine training in undergraduate medical education: a review and critique of the literature published 2006-2011. Acad Med 2013;88(7):1022–8.

14. Green ML. Graduate medical education training in clinical epidemiology, critical appraisal, and evidence-based medicine: a critical review of curricula. Acad Med 1999;74(6):686–94.

15. Coomarasamy A, Taylor R, Khan KS. A systematic review of postgraduate teaching in evidence-based medicine and critical appraisal. Med Teach 2003;25(1):77–81.

16. United States Medical Licensing Examination ®. Available at: https://www.usmle.org/. Accessed April 22, 2019.

17. Alguire PC. A review of journal clubs in postgraduate medical education. J Gen Intern Med 1998;13(5):347–53.

18. Horsley T, Hyde C, Santesso N, et al. Teaching critical appraisal skills in healthcare settings. Cochrane Database Syst Rev 2011;(11). https://doi.org/10.1002/14651858.CD001270.pub2.

19. American College of Rheumatology. 2018 ACR/ARHP Annual meeting. ACR - 2018 ACR/ARHP Annual meeting 2018. Available at: https://acr.confex.com/acr/2018/meetingapp.cgi/Index/Track ~ Clinical and Translational Research. Accessed March 22, 2019.

20. American College of Rheumatology. Rheum4Science module 4 - data and Distributions 2019. Available at: https://www.rheumatology.org/Learning-Center/Educational-Activities/View/ID/952. Accessed March 4, 2019.

21. Bordage G. Conceptual frameworks to illuminate and magnify. Med Educ 2009; 43(4):312–9.

22. Taylor DCM, Hamdy H. Adult learning theories: implications for learning and teaching in medical education: AMEE Guide No. 83. Med Teach 2013;35(11): e1561–72.

23. Roediger HL III, Butler AC. The critical role of retrieval practice in long-term retention. Trends Cogn Sci 2011;15(1):8.

24. Karpicke JD, Grimaldi PJ. Retrieval-based learning: a perspective for enhancing meaningful learning. Educ Psychol Rev 2012;24:401–18. https://doi.org/10.1007/s10648-012-9202-2.

25. Roediger HL III, Karpicke JD. The power of testing memory: basic research and implications for educational practice. Perspect Psychol Sci 2006;1(3): 181–210.

26. Karpicke JD. Retrieval-based learning: a decade of progress. In: Cognitive Psychology of Memory, Vol. 2 of Learning and Memory: A Comprehensive Reference. 2017. Available at: https://doi.org/10.1016/B978-0-12-809324-5.21055-9. Accessed February 27, 2019.

27. National Academies of Sciences E. How People Learn II: Learners, Contexts, and Cultures.; 2018. https://doi.org/10.17226/24783.
28. Schell JA. Insights from the science of learning can inform evidence-based implementation of peer instruction. Front Educ 2018;3:13. https://doi.org/10.3389/feduc.2018.00033.
29. Keengwe J, Onchwari G. Handbook of Research on Learner-Centered Pedagogy in Teacher Education and Professional Development. IGI Global. 2001. Available at: https://www.igi-global.com/book/handbook-research-learner-centered-pedagogy/152429. Accessed April 22, 2019.
30. Karpicke JD, Aue WR. The testing effect is alive and well with complex materials. Educ Psychol Rev 2015;27(2):317–26.
31. Chan JC. When does retrieval induce forgetting and when does it induce facilitation? Implications for retrieval inhibition, testing effect, and text processing - ScienceDirect. J Mem Lang 2009;61(2):153–70.
32. Butler AC, Godbole N, Marsh EJ. Explanation feedback is better than correct answer feedback for promoting transfer of learning. J Educ Psychol 2013; 105(2):290–8.
33. Schell J, Butler AC. Insights from the science of learning: understanding why peer instruction is effective can inform implementation. In: Vol 3. Frontiers; 2018:33.
34. Butler AC, Roediger HL. Feedback enhances the positive effects and reduces the negative effects of multiple-choice testing. Mem Cognit 2008;36(3):604–16.
35. Ryan RM, Deci EL. Self-determination theory and the facilitation of intrinsic motivation, social development, and well-being. Am Psychol 2000;55(1):68–78.
36. Deci EL, Vallerand RJ, Pelletier LG, et al. Motivation and education: the self-determination perspective. Educ Psychol 1991;26(3–4):325–46.
37. Deci EL, Ryan RM. The "what" and "why" of goal pursuits: human needs and the self-determination of behavior. Psychol Inq 2000;11(4):227–68.
38. Ryan RM, Vallerand RJ, Deci EL. Intrinsic motivation and self-determination in human behavior. In: Straub WF, Williams JM, editors. Cognitive sports psychology. New York: Sports Science Associates; 1984. p. 231–42. Available at: https://www.researchgate.net/publication/233896840_Intrinsic_Motivation_and_Self-Determination_in_Human_Behavior. Accessed March 4, 2019.
39. Multon KD, Brown SD, Lent RW. Relation of self-efficacy beliefs to academic outcomes: a meta-analytic investigation. J Couns Psychol 1991;38(1):30–8.
40. Phillips JC, Russell RK. Research self-efficacy, the research training environment, and research productivity among graduate students in counseling psychology. Couns Psychol 1994;22(4):628–41.
41. Lave J, Wenger E. Situated Learning: Legitimate Peripheral Participation. Cambridge university press; 1991.
42. Barab SA, Barnett M, Squire K. Developing an empirical account of a community of practice: characterizing the essential tensions. J Learn Sci 2002;11(4):489–542.
43. Cruess R, Cruess S, Steinert Y. Medicine as a community of practice: implications for medical education. Acad Med 2018;93(2):185–91.
44. Land R, Meyer J, Smith J. Threshold concepts within the disciplines. Rotterdam/Taipei: Sense Publishers; 2008.
45. Bernstein BB. Pedagogy, symbolic Control, and identity: theory, research, critique. Lanham, MD: Rowman & Littlefield; 2000.
46. Aizer J, Schell J, Collins C, et al. Development and implementation of a question-based tool promoting learning of relevant epidemiology and biostatistics in rheumatology: the critical literature assessment skills support - rheumatology (CLASS-

Rheum) pilot [abstract]. Arthritis Rheumatol 2016;68(suppl 10). Available at: https://acrabstracts.org/abstract/development-and-implementation-of-a-question-based-tool-promoting-learning-of-relevant-epidemiology-and-biostatistics-in-rheumatology-the-critical-literature-assessment-skills-support-rheumatology/. Accessed March 4, 2019.

47. Paniagua MA, Swygert KA, editors. Constructing written test questions for the basic and clinical sciences. 4th edition. Philadelphia: National Board of Medical Examiners; 2016.

48. Schell J. How to transform learning-with teaching. Lead Learn; 2012. p. 3–6.

49. Schuller MC, DaRosa DA, Crandall ML. Using just-in-time teaching and peer instruction in a residency program's core curriculum: enhancing satisfaction, engagement, and retention. Acad Med 2015;90(3):384–91.

50. Schell JA, Porter JR. Applying the science of learning to classroom teaching: the critical importance of aligning learning with testing. J Food Sci Educ 2018;17(2):36–41.

51. Miller K, Schell J, Ho A, et al. Response switching and self-efficacy in Peer Instruction classrooms. 2015:8.

52. Mazur E. Peer instruction: a user's manual. In: Short G, Harten U, editors. Pearson; 1996.

53. Müller MG, Araujo IS, Veit EA, et al. A literature review on the implementation of Peer Instruction interactive teaching method (1991 to 2015). Rev Bras Ensino Física 2017;39(3).

54. Mandl LA, Schell J, Torralba K, et al. The CLASS-rheum (critical literature assessment skills support – rheumatology) question-based tool is associated with sustained improvement in knowledge of relevant epidemiology and biostatistics in rheumatology fellows [abstract]. Arthritis Rheumatol 2017;69(suppl 10). Available at: https://acrabstracts.org/abstract/the-class-rheum-critical-literature-assessment-skills-support-rheumatology-question-based-tool-is-associated-with-sustained-improvement-in-knowledge-of-relevant-epidemiology-and-biostatist/. Accessed March 4, 2019.

55. Taylor R, Reeves B, Ewings P, et al. A systematic review of the effectiveness of critical appraisal skills training for clinicians. Med Educ 2000;34(2):120–5.

56. Windish DM, Huot SJ, Green ML. Medicine residents' understanding of the biostatistics and results in the medical literature. JAMA 2007;298(9):1010–22.

57. Young JM, Glasziou P, Ward JE. General Practitioners' self ratings of skills in evidence based medicine: validation study. BMJ 2002;324:950–1.

58. McMahon GT, Skochelak SE. Evolution of continuing medical education: promoting innovation through regulatory alignment. JAMA 2018;319(6):545–6.

59. McMahon GT. Inspiring curiosity and restoring humility: the evolution of competency-based continuing medical education. Acad Med 2018;93(12):1757–9.

60. Collins C, Sufka P, Bhana S, et al. Amigues I. #RheumJC. #RheumJC. Available at: https://rheumjc.com/. Accessed February 27, 2019.

61. Collins C, Sufka P, Hausmann JS, et al. #Rheumjc: development, implementation and analysis of an international twitter-based rheumatology journal club [abstract]. Arthritis Rheumatol. 67(suppl 10). Available at: https://acrabstracts.org/abstract/rheumjcdevelopment-implementation-and-analysis-of-an-international-twitter-based-rheumatologyjournal-club/. Accessed February 27, 2019.

62. Amigues I, Sufka P, Bhana S, et al. #Rheumjc: Impact of Invited Authors on a Twitter Based Rheumatology Journal Club [abstract]. Arthritis Rheumatol. 68(suppl 10). Available at: https://acrabstracts.org/abstract/rheumjc-impact-of-invited-authors-on-a-twitter-basedrheumatology-journal-club/. Accessed February 27, 2019.

63. Collins C, Campos J, Isabelle A, et al. #rheumjc: 3 year analysis of a twitter based rheumatology journal club [AB1385]. Ann Rheum Dis 2018;77(S2):1777.
64. Goldstein A, Venker E, Weng C. Evidence appraisal: a scoping review, conceptual framework, and research agenda. J Am Med Inform Assoc 2017;24(6):1192–203.
65. Chan K, Cheung G, Wan K, et al. Synthesizing technology adoption and learners' approaches towards Active Learning in Higher Education. 2015;13(6):10.

Mind the Gap
Improving Care in Pediatric-to-Adult Rheumatology Transition Through Education

Rebecca E. Sadun, MD, PhD

KEYWORDS

- Adolescent and young adult • Youth with special health care needs
- Health care transition and transfer • Rheumatology fellowship curriculum
- Graduate medical education

KEY POINTS

- Young adults (aged 18–25) have worse health outcomes than patients 12 to 17 or 26 to 34, and morbidity and mortality increase when young adults transfer from pediatric to adult care.
- Rheumatology fellows in the Unites States are expected to "maintain appropriate continuity during transitions of care, including from pediatric to adult rheumatology care."
- The American College of Rheumatology Transition Toolkit and Got Transition offer point-of-care resources to support caring for adolescents and young adult rheumatology patients.
- Curricula in young adult transition best practices help adult rheumatology fellows develop increased confidence and competence in caring for young adult patients.
- Experiential learning methodologies are especially well suited to transforming how physicians help adolescent and young adult patients succeed within the adult health care system.

INTRODUCTION

Each year thousands of young adults with rheumatic diseases are advised to transfer from the care of a pediatric rheumatologist to that of a rheumatologist who is specialized in the care of adult patients. For some young adults, this transfer of care entails no more than walking down a hall, whereas for others it requires changing health care systems. Whether the distance traveled is short or far, there can exist a chasm

Disclosure: The author is the recipient of a Clinician Scholar Educator Award from the Rheumatology Research Foundation to complete a project that entails developing a transition curriculum for rheumatology fellows.
Adult and Pediatric Rheumatology, Duke University Medical Center, 200 Trent Drive, Durham, NC 27710, USA
E-mail address: Rebecca.Sadun@duke.edu

between pediatric and adult specialty services, and many young adult patients with chronic illness fail to establish with an adult provider. More specifically, an estimated 50% of pediatric rheumatology patients fall out of care at this juncture.[1–3]

Over the last 20 years, the medical profession has identified many of the challenges that contribute to this disruption in care, leading to new quality improvement measures and education interventions that can help young adults and their families "aimed at helping" so as to integrate into adult rheumatology care more successfully. Indeed, there are now several published sets of recommendations that guide rheumatologists in how to successfully transition and transfer young adult patients with pediatric-onset rheumatic diseases.[4–6] Currently, however, trainees in all fields of medicine report receiving minimal formal training in transition and transfer best practices as well as limited role modeling.[7] Furthermore, a recent national survey estimated that nearly half of the adult rheumatologists practicing in the United States feel uncomfortable caring for young adults with a childhood-onset rheumatic disease.[8]

In 2014, US internal medicine subspecialty programs, including rheumatology fellowships, implemented a set of 23 reporting milestones for trainees. These milestones define the skills that fellows should demonstrate before graduation as well as "aspirational" goals. One milestone states that a fellow "transitions patients effectively within and across health delivery systems" (System Based Practice Reporting Milestone 4) and another stipulates that a fellow "communicates effectively in interprofessional teams ... [which includes] communication with other health care providers in order to maintain appropriate continuity during transitions of care, including from pediatric to adult rheumatology care" (Interpersonal and Communication Skills Reporting Milestone 2).[9,10] In addition, one of the 14 rheumatology entrustable professional activities (EPAs) was set forth as "Effectively communicate and manage transitions of care with other healthcare providers."[9,11] There are not, however, any guidelines on how to help fellows achieve proficiency in these arenas, raising the question of *how* we train the next generation of rheumatologists so that we can entrust them with the care of young adult rheumatology patients.

As more is learned about transition and transfer best practices, rheumatologists in training as well as those in practice must learn how to implement new transition guidelines and use new evidence-based transition tools. Through the cultivation and creation of curricula and relevant educational opportunities, adult and pediatric rheumatologists can develop the attitudes, knowledge, and skills that are critical to the delivery of excellent transitional care:

1. Attitudes: appreciation of the challenges faced by adolescents and young adults (AYA) and their families before, during, and after transfer; recognition of the role physicians play in perpetuating versus mitigating these challenges
2. Knowledge: familiarity with transition best practices and rheumatology-specific guidelines for transition and transfer; understanding of the specific factors that contribute to AYA vulnerability and methodologies for addressing this vulnerability
3. Skills: development of effective communication techniques for working with AYA patients and their families; skill in the application of existing transition and transfer tools

This article reviews the literature on teaching physicians to help young adults with the transition and transfer process and discusses a broad swath of rheumatology transition interventions. Finally, this article reviews in-depth existing rheumatology-specific transition curricula as well as other education opportunities grounded in learning theory.

THE ROOTS OF THE PROBLEM

Numerous factors contribute to the disruption or disintegration of care that occurs when young adults transfer from pediatric to adult care.[12] Many of these problems are tied to cultural differences between pediatric and adult health care systems,[13–16] whereas others are related to challenges inherent in caring for AYA, including emotional or irrational behavior owing to a still-developing prefrontal cortex,[17–19] low rates of medication adherence,[20,21] high rates of depression,[22–24] high-risk or self-destructive behaviors,[25,26] frequent relocation for school or work,[27] and limited financial stability.[28]

There are many additional challenges working with AYA patients. This age group often prioritizes short-term interests ahead of health, while being minimally influenced by future-oriented consequences. In addition, young adulthood is characterized by many changes over a short period of time (eg, starting or stopping school, changing jobs); transfer of care is often precipitated by changes such as the patient moving (for work or for school), losing insurance coverage (eg, aging out of Medicaid), or other major life events (eg, pregnancy), any one of which can place the patient in an unfamiliar and sometimes precarious circumstance. Furthermore, effective communication with AYA patients often requires specific skills, such as requesting that a parent leave the room before asking sensitive social history questions and exploring the many dimensions of an adolescent social history (eg, education/employment goals and peer influences); graduates of internal medicine training programs are rarely practiced in these dialogues.

Beyond these factors intrinsic to AYA patients, cultural differences between pediatric and adult health care systems contribute to disruptions during the transfer between the two systems. For example, pediatric providers are often more apt to "hand-hold" and to interact with parents "on behalf of" a pediatric patient, whereas the adult health care system is more likely to hold the young adult patient responsible for self-management. Parents accompanying their AYA child to an adult clinic visit may feel alienated by their sudden lack of involvement with adult health care teams, which may lead them to undermine (intentionally or unintentionally) the development of an effective working relationship between a young adult child and the adult-oriented rheumatologist.

In addition, pediatric patients and their parents are used to a health care system that is more lenient toward appointment no-shows or tardiness, with pediatric clinics often initiating the rescheduling of appointments after missed appointments. After transfer, patients and families may be offended by the enforcement of stricter rules and be unprepared for the loss of safety nets. Whereas pediatric clinics may be more willing to accommodate urgent visit requests, young adults may feel put off because adult clinics are less accommodating and more likely to prescribe a steroid taper over the telephone rather than bring the patient in for a visit.

As opposed to adult clinics, many pediatric clinics have on-site ancillary staff, such as social workers, who can help patients stay engaged in care. In addition, adult clinic appointments are often briefer; pediatric appointments in the United States are generally 30 minutes as compared with the 15 minutes slated for many adult rheumatology return visits. In this context, AYA patients and their parents may feel that the adult provider is hurried. Moreover, because of shorter visits, it can be more challenging for an adult provider to uncover many of the common the psychosocial issues that interfere with medical care (eg, lack of transportation and other financial challenges, differing cultural beliefs regarding medication, or common mental health problems like depression that can interfere with adherence).

In addition, common medical practices can vary between pediatric and adult clinics. For example, pediatric lupus patients may be more routinely screened with echocardiographs, pediatric providers are more likely to use intravenous pulse steroids, and medication dosing is more commonly weight based in pediatrics. After transfer, AYA patients and their families may feel threatened when a new adult provider follows different guidelines or abides by different dosing protocols. Even though these practice changes may be routine and evidence based in adult rheumatology, families who saw a pediatric rheumatologist's practice as "the right way" of providing care may see any deviation from this course of action as "the wrong way" to practice. Furthermore, it is unfortunate that in many cases a "hidden curriculum" has taught AYA patients and their parents to fear adult health care. Indeed, use of phrases that carry a negative connotation, such as, "don't worry, we won't *make you* transfer until you graduate from college," may communicate pediatric provider distrust of adult care.

In addition to these many cultural challenges, transfer to adult care is fraught with technical challenges, such as the fact that medical records may fail to follow the patient, or unorganized records of little use are sent. The adult rheumatologist is therefore at a disadvantage in caring for the young adult patient with a complex past medical history. In this case, patients and families may be quick to fault an adult provider for not knowing the patient as well as did the transferring pediatric provider. Similarly, during a first visit with an adult rheumatologist, patients and families are prone to unfavorably compare the new, "getting to know one another" interaction with the prior long-standing, close-knit relationship of trust.

Because few rheumatologists have experience in both the pediatric and the adult aspects of the health care system, providers do not have first-hand knowledge of these enumerated cultural differences; as such, it can be hard for providers to describe these differences to families or otherwise help patients navigate the "culture shock." To address this unmet need, Got Transitions has developed a handout for AYA patients and their families, delineating many of the common differences between pediatric and adult care.[29]

Unfortunately, despite the rich recent literature in transition, we do not currently know the relative importance of the above-mentioned challenges and do not have a way to identify, for a given adolescent patient, which factors pose the greatest threat. Nevertheless, from the body of evidence that exists regarding the perils of young adult transition in rheumatology, and drawing upon what medicine has learned from tackling other challenging patient transitions (such as from the hospital to the outpatient setting), four critical areas can be identified as targets for educational interventions aimed at improving young adult transition in rheumatology care:

1. Training pediatric rheumatology providers to prepare adolescent patients and their families for transfer by promoting self-management, transitioning to an adult model of care for late adolescent patients seen in pediatric care, and providing families with realistic expectations of adult care, including common cultural differences to be anticipated
2. Enhancing communication between pediatric rheumatologists and adult rheumatologists, so that critical patient-specific information (psychosocial, in addition to biological) is relayed by or before the time of transfer
3. Training adult rheumatologists to recognize and effectively manage both age-specific challenges and challenges related to cultural differences between pediatric and adult care systems

4. Creating systems, including but not limited to transition clinics and quality improvement practices, surrounding the use of readiness assessment measures and transfer registries to support patients before, during, and after transfer

TRANSITION GUIDELINES IN RHEUMATOLOGY

A 2015 consensus statement from the Spanish Society of Pediatric Rheumatology used a Delphi process to establish 18 recommendations for improving transitional care, including training pediatric rheumatologists and other health care professionals in transitional care best practices and models of care.[6] In 2017, a European-wide panel of pediatric rheumatologists and nephrologists developed a set of recommendations for the transition and transfer of patients with pediatric-onset systemic lupus erythematosus, advising that adolescent patients be supported through transition and transfer while also advocating for concerted efforts to develop adolescents' self-management skills, including special attention to the problem of therapeutic nonadherence.[5]

Notably, in 2016 the European League Against Rheumatism (EULAR) and the Paediatric Rheumatology European Society (PReS) jointly published transition recommendations for AYA with pediatric-onset rheumatic diseases based on the work of an expert panel and refined by input from 200 European adult and pediatric rheumatology specialists.[4] This report offered 12 recommendations, including the guiding principles, that (1) every rheumatology service have a written transition policy, (2) transition discussions begin in early adolescence, and (3) transitional care be individualized, based on the needs and abilities of patients and their families. The report also recommended that rheumatology care of the adolescent and young adult patient address the medical, psychosocial, and educational/vocational needs of patients. Their definition of "holistic care" deviates from customary adult clinic practices in several arenas, including recommendations that adult providers borrow key strategies from adolescent medicine, such as identifying a young adult patient's needs and risks through a social history that considers Home, Education, peer Activities, Drugs, Sex, and Suicide/depression (HEADSS).[30] In addition, these guidelines recommend that a transfer document should accompany transferring patients, that there should be direct communication between the pediatric and adult rheumatologists both before and after transfer, and that there be a designated transition coordinator.

Two surveys established pediatric rheumatologists' baseline transition practices before the dissemination of the EULAR/PReS recommendations. In a 2008 survey of 158 pediatric rheumatologists in Canada and the United States, only 6% said they provided young adults assistance in creating individualized health care transition plans.[31] In 2016, 121 pediatric rheumatologists from 22 European countries responded to a similar survey, revealing that only 33% had a written transition policy, and less than 10% used a specific assessment tool to identify readiness for transfer.[32] Interestingly, 64% reported having a designated staff member primarily responsible for coordinating the transition process, which likely exceeds current US practices.

Shortly following the EULAR/PReS publication and 2 years after the American College of Rheumatology (ACR) released a "Pediatric to Adult Care Transition Toolkit,"[33] the Canadian/US survey was repeated, revealing that 17% of providers had a written transition policy, 31% of providers used the ACR Toolkit, and 37% of providers reported consistently addressing health care transition with their patients.[34] Although this 2018 study represents some improvements from the 2008 study, there is considerable room for improvement at a national level.

ENTER GOT TRANSITION

In response to the need for widespread implementation of foundational transition and transfer best practices, the Got Transition Center for Health Care Transition Improvement was developed as a cooperative agreement between the US Maternal and Child Health Bureau and The National Alliance to Advance Adolescent Health. The program's aim is "to improve transition from pediatric to adult health care through the use of new and innovative strategies for health professionals and youth and families."[35]

Got Transition developed the Six Core Elements of Health Care Transition 2.0, which "defines the basic components of healthcare transition support … [to] include establishing a policy, tracking progress, administering transition readiness assessments, planning for adult care, transferring, and integrating into an adult practice."[36] Through the Six Core Elements, it becomes possible for providers, practices, and health systems to evaluate the transition services they provide patients and families, while facilitating quality improvement work in each of the 6 arenas.[37] At a health system level, it becomes possible to measure and track transfer outcomes.[38] Ultimately, it will be possible to evaluate transition within the framework of the canonical "triple aim": the patient experience of care, the health of the population, and the cost of health care.[39]

Importantly, Got Transition's website (https://www.gottransition.org/) provides patients, parents, and providers with access to transition tools and resources. Of course, a tool is only as good as its user, and in the case of transition tools, the rheumatologist is sometimes unaware of why the tools are important, where to find the tools, and how to use the tools. For the tools to have broad impact, rheumatologists must be trained in their purpose as well as their application, including the appropriate setting for utilization and appropriate interpretation of the data obtained.

The Got Transition team, working in conjunction with the American Academy of Pediatrics, the American Academy of Family Physicians, and the American College of Physicians, published the 2018 clinical report on supporting health care transition,[40] which serves as an update to the seminal 2011 clinical report.[41] The 2018 report "provides practice-based quality improvement guidance on key elements of transition planning, transfer, and integration into adult care for all youth and young adults." In addition to offering strong evidence for the need for structured transition support and explaining the implementation of the Six Core Elements, the report touches on continuing medical education (CME) and other training opportunities as well as outlining mechanisms for reimbursement for the clinical provision of health care transition services.

NONRHEUMATOLOGY-SPECIFIC TRANSITION CURRICULA

In response to the need for transition education materials, several CME courses have been developed, including by the Society for Adolescent Health and Medicine[42,43] and by the Illinois Chapter of the American Academy of Pediatrics, with modules intended for general pediatricians, internists, or family practitioners.[44] In addition, a transition case of a 15-year-old with inflammatory bowel disease was published in MedEd Portal and can be used to stimulate case-based discussion about transition.[45] Unfortunately, even while some residencies are developing pilot curricula to teach transition,[46,47] as of 2019 there can be no expectations that fellows entering rheumatology programs will have developed transition skills during residency given that there are presently no transition-related residency requirements in pediatrics, internal medicine, medicine/pediatrics, or family medicine.[48]

Recently, expert opinion was sought from 56 international health care transition professionals via a modified Delphi process that identified education goals for residents training in primary care.[49] The 5 overarching educational goals agreed upon were for residents to:

1. Understand the transition from pediatric to adult health care (8 subobjectives)
2. Understand insurance policies and social services (4 subobjectives)
3. Consider developmental and psychosocial needs (12 subobjectives)
4. Address educational and vocational needs (4 subobjectives)
5. Improve health care systems for youth with special health care needs (4 subobjectives)

Of the 32 specific objectives identified by this group, several were skills based, including that each resident should be able to perform a complete history and physical in AYA with physical and/or intellectual disabilities; communicate and coordinate effectively around handoffs in health care transition between pediatric and adult providers; demonstrate the ability to work as an effective member of an interprofessional team to support transitioning AYA; develop and update transition care plans, address patients' decision-making status and self-management skills; apply effective coding and billing practice for health care transition services; and use a transfer package, inclusive of a readiness assessment, medical summary, emergency care plan, and any needed legal documents.

Because transition is often viewed as a "problem that pediatricians need to address prior to transfer," several pediatrics residency programs have developed transition curricula. For example, faculty at the pediatrics residency program at the University of South Florida developed a transition curriculum for all of their pediatrics and medicine-pediatrics residents using a behavior change framework.[46] Training included a 45-minute lecture about guidelines in health care transition that was reinforced through the development and dissemination of several electronic health record transition tools to assess AYA patients' self-management skills. Analysis of the pretests and posttests demonstrated that the intervention increased residents' knowledge regarding transition best practices in addition to improving residents' confidence in developing a transition plan for youth with special health care needs.

In light of the fact that most patients transfer to adult care before they have mastered self-management or outgrown the involvement of their parents in their medical care, several transition curricula have recently been developed for internal medicine residents and/or residents in other nonpediatric specialties. One innovative approach to educating residents involved having residents from pediatrics, internal medicine, and medicine-pediatrics work alongside each other, in dyads, in a transition clinic. This clinic provided care to patients aged 16 to 26 with chronic medical illnesses, neurodevelopmental disorders, or mental health diagnoses that interfered with patients' ability to progress along expected transition milestones.[47] Residents learned from each other about different approaches to the care of adolescent and young adult patients, while also providing trainees with the opportunity to observe a social worker conduct transition readiness assessments. In addition, the clinic incorporated young adult peer coaches and parent navigators, along with attending physicians in pediatrics, adolescent medicine, internal medicine, psychiatry, and neurology, providing residents a chance to observe and engage in team-based, interdisciplinary care. After rotating through the clinic, residents from each field reported increased preparedness in counseling young adults and families. Internal medicine residents also felt more prepared to receive young adults into their care, and all residents felt better able to communicate with physicians from a different specialty (ie, pediatrics residents felt more comfortable speaking to internal medicine residents, and vice versa). Additional education research is needed to show whether this transition experience changes participating trainees' behaviors with AYA patients and whether changes in provider transition behaviors result in better health outcomes for AYA patients.

CURRICULA IN RHEUMATOLOGY

At the present time, there is very limited published literature on rheumatology-specific educational interventions on transition. In 1 study, a 1-hour workshop for adult rheumatology fellows enhanced learner confidence in key transition skills and was associated with higher scores on a transition station in an objective standardized clinical examination (OSCE).[50] The workshop highlighted the struggles faced by transferring patients and their families as well as the morbidity and mortality associated with transfer, while focusing on providing participants with strategies for working with young adults and their parents.

The content of the workshop included the difference between "transition" (the process of developing the skills needed to manage one's own health care) and "transfer" (the act of moving from pediatric to adult care),[1–4,51,52] cultural differences between pediatric and adult health care systems,[13–16,40,53] setting expectations related to these differences, measurement of young adults' self-management,[54–57] common barriers to care for young adults,[12] the insurance landscape for young adults,[58] the HEADSS model for adolescent social history,[59] asking a parent to leave the room,[60] and an introduction to the ACR's transition tools.[33]

As illustrated in **Fig. 1**, this 1-hour workshop was offered to 19 adult rheumatology fellows from 5 institutions, each of whom completed a preassessment and postassessment of confidence in their ability to carry out an array of tasks related to working with young adult patients. Fellows were also evaluated by an OSCE station designed to test fellows' abilities to interact with a young adult lupus patient and her mother for a first adult visit following transfer from pediatric rheumatology. Results from the workshop evaluation showed that fellows' confidence increased significantly in 8 of 10 domains, and fellows who participated in the workshop before the OSCE demonstrated greater competence in the following 3 arenas: (1) providing the patient and family with clear expectations of adult-oriented care, including the implications of HIPAA; (2)

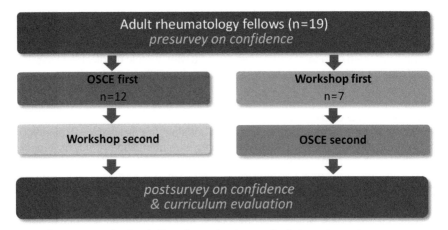

Fig. 1. Objective standardized clinical examination study design schematic.

eliciting the history primarily from the AYA patient, while using the parent for corroboration; and (3) performing a confidential adolescent social history, including asking the parent to leave.

A longer version of this curriculum was offered in the format of a 2-hour workshop at the 2018 Annual Meeting of the American College of Rheumatology, led by 3 rheumatologists dually trained in adult and pediatric rheumatology.[61] In addition to the topics discussed above, the 2-hour format included a session on the neuroscience of AYA, considerations specific to caring for "millennials," and training on the legal ramifications of the HIPAA, whereby a patient 18 or older must provide consent for medical information to be shared with or in front of parents, including for parents to remain in the room during any part of a clinic visit.

Participants were also introduced to multiple tools from Got Transitions[36] and to 2 mnemonics, one designed to provide a model for communication between pediatric and adult providers at the time of transfer (**Box 1**), and the other a model for welcoming a young adult patient and family to a first visit in adult care (**Box 2**).[15] In addition, participants were paired up so that they had the opportunity to practice 2 important skills: (1) asking a parent to leave the room and (2) helping a young adult set his or her own transition goals.

To illustrate effective and ineffective ways of managing the physician-patient-parent triad, facilitators interviewed a young adult actor with a second actor playing the role of her mother. In the first scenario, the physician let the parent dominate the interview, answering all of the physician's questions while the young adult played on a cell phone; in the next scenario, the physician insisted that the young adult answer all interview questions, unintentionally alienating the parent by repeatedly silencing her. In the final scenario, the physician began the interview by setting the expectation that the young adult should answer each question herself, after which the physician would turn to the parent to see if she had anything to add; this scenario highlighted how the physician can build rapport with a young adult patient, while enabling the parent to fulfill a meaningful but unobtrusive role.

There were not enough workshop participants to allow for comparative statistics; however, a review of participants' postsurveys revealed that the most meaningful workshop takeaway lessons were getting comfortable with asking a parent to leave the room, learning how to use self-management tools to enhance efficiency, and

---

Box 1
TRANSFERS

Communication between paediatric and adult rheumatology providers before the first adult visit, as a supplement to a written medical summary.
- Treatment history.
- Recent complications. Recent medication changes and so on.
- Adherence challenges (including assessment of root causes).
- Needs (eg, referral to adult nephrology, establish with mental health provider).
- Social history and Social challenges.
- Financial/insurance challenges.
- Emotional or intellectual challenges.
- Reasons this a good (or precarious) time for transfer.
- Summary of patient characteristics (eg, favourite activities, academic interests, professional goals, personal values).

From Sadun RE, Schanberg LE. Transition and transfer of the patient with paediatric-onset lupus: a practical approach for paediatric and adult rheumatology practices. Lupus Sci Med. 2018;5(1):e000282; with permission.

Box 2
WELCOME

Steps for the adult rheumatology provider to take when a patient arrives from paediatric care.
- Welcome and congratulate the patient on graduating to adult care.
- Explain key similarities and differences (medical and structural) between paediatric and adult care.
- Let patient and parents know their respective roles (eg, the patient answers questions first, after which input from parent welcomed).
- Communication ongoing with the paediatric provider reassure he patient you are in touch as needed.
- Opportunity for the patient and parents to ask questions about the new clinic (before beginning medical aspects of the visit).
- Minimise medical changes during first adult clinic visit.
- Expectations supportively convey expectations of the patient and parents (eg, arrive 10 minutes prior to your appointment).

From Sadun RE, Schanberg LE. Transition and transfer of the patient with paediatric-onset lupus: a practical approach for paediatric and adult rheumatology practices. Lupus Sci Med. 2018;5(1):e000282; with permission.

---

developing communication strategies for conversations between pediatric and adult providers. In addition, workshop participants were asked if there was anything they planned to start doing after the workshop that they had not planned to do before the workshop. Concrete goals identified by workshop participants included creating a clinic transition policy, tracking self-management skills during clinic visits, and developing lines of ongoing communication between pediatric and adult rheumatologists to facilitate shared management of complex patients.

THEORY-BASED TRANSITION EDUCATION OPPORTUNITIES

The goal of transition education is to transform how providers approach AYA patients, which is likely to require more than transmission of information through a traditional lecture. Indeed, a survey of primary care residents identified that residents prefer a longitudinal transition curriculum that is inclusive of clinical experiences and case discussions.[62] Adult learning theory suggests that experiential learning can enhance the impact that transition training has on the ways in which rheumatologists, pediatric and adult, address the needs of AYA patients. Kolb[63] outlined 4 stages of experiential learning, all of which can be applied to transition education as illustrated by the examples in **Table 1**. Indeed, in keeping with the central role that experiential learning plays in adult learning theory, new curricula in transition should incorporate (1) a case-based approach (which can take the form of individual and group analysis of participants' previous clinical experiences with AYA patients), (2) discussion of and practice with transition vignettes (inclusive of role-playing opportunities), (3) formative use of transition OSCEs (inclusive of the opportunity to self-reflect and to receive feedback on one's performance), and (4) prospective application of transitional care techniques in real clinical settings (inclusive of the opportunity to reflect on their experiences and receive feedback, either direct or indirect, on strengths and weaknesses).

Transition vignettes are likely to be impactful because they are problem centered, are task oriented, draw on learners' experiences, and provide a basis for internal motivation to learn.[64] From vignettes, learners can begin to develop "illness scripts" or "clinical case categories," such as "this is a case of a young adult with poor self-management due to low self-efficacy" or "this is a case of a young adult with poor self-management due to low assigned importance." Learners can take these illness

Table 1 Application of Kolb's Experiential Learning Cycle to transition training	
Concrete experience	*Definition:* Adults learn best through real or realistic scenarios that demonstrate cause-and-effect relationships. Powerful experiences that evoke strong emotional responses strengthen learning *Application:* Through real cases and realistic vignettes about AYA patients struggling with transition, learners can be guided to identify ways in which departure from transition best practices result in unfortunate transfer outcomes (such as a clinical flare due to an AYA patient coming off medication, due to the patient falling out of adult care, due to missed opportunities during the transfer visit). This can be done through informal discussion or more formally with root cause analysis tools
Reflective observation	*Definition:* Adults learn through reflecting on their own experiences and having the opportunity to independently connect new concepts to previous experiences *Application:* Learners can be encouraged to reflect on their own actions with AYA patients, using either actual patient encounters from a recent clinical setting or performance during a transition-focused AYA OSCE case. Learners can be asked what they or others have done well with AYA patients, and where transition support could be strengthened
Abstract conceptualization	*Definition:* Out of reflections, learners abstract or decode general concepts, generalizing them so that they can be applicable to scenarios that extend beyond the one upon which they have reflected *Application:* In the same settings outlined above, learners can be asked how additional transition best practices could have been applied to specific cases (real or simulated)
Active experimentation	*Definition:* The application of generalized concepts enables learners to "learn by doing." This often entails experimentation and practice, first in safe learning environments and then in authentic settings *Application:* Through the development of transition vignettes, learners can practice core transition concepts and skills in role-playing scenarios that allow them to try different approaches and establish the communication strategies that work best for them. For example, a rheumatology fellow might practice asking a parent to leave the room multiple times in a role-playing scenario before constructing a "script" that feels comfortable enough for him/her to use and refine it in clinical practice

scripts a step further by identifying the most appropriate communication technique or transition tool for a given illness script, such as using motivational interviewing techniques to address the basis of an AYA patient's poor self-management.

Furthermore, in order to have a sustained impact on rheumatologists' future behaviors, a case-based curriculum should be designed to incorporate the 3 components of transformational learning: identification of a dilemma, establishment of personal relevance, and critical thinking.[65] Creative educational exercises in which such transformational learning could take place emphasize dialogue and collaborative learning that also involves critically exploring diverse viewpoints. For example:

- Pediatric trainees observing AYA clinical encounters in the adult clinics, and vice versa with adult trainees observing young adult care in the pediatric clinical setting (experiential learning)

- Adult and/or pediatric trainees observing a transfer by attending both the last pediatric rheumatology clinic visit and that patient's first 2 adult visits (process reflection)
- Pediatric and adult rheumatology trainees meeting in person to discuss a transferring patient and collaborating on a transfer plan that best addresses the transition needs (premise reflection)
- Pediatric and adult divisions, when coexisting at a single institution, jointly discussing young adult cases, touching on both the medical care aspects and the transitional care aspects of the patients' cases; cases can be presented either as current clinical conundrums the 2 divisions need to work together to address or as morbidity and mortality cases, in response to which the divisions can work together to identify failures as well as system-wide opportunities for improvement (reflection-"on"-action)
- Transitional care reflection logs, in which rheumatologists prospectively document application of transition best practices as well as missed opportunities (reflection-"in"-action)
- Using the 6 quality improvement initiatives in Got Transition Six Core Elements of Health Care Transition 2.0 as a model for teaching the principles of quality improvement within a residency or fellowship training program[66]

SUMMARY

Young adults account for 5% to 10% of rheumatology patients, a small enough percentage for providers to feel uncomfortable caring for these patients,[8,67] and yet more than enough patients to warrant system-wide quality improvement and education interventions to ensure these patients receive high quality care. It is critical for rheumatologists to recognize the many ways in which young adults differ from older patients: different biology, different psychology, and different family ecology. Beyond that, patients transferring from pediatric rheumatology come with added expectations and fears that can bring unfamiliar and unwanted challenges to the physician-patient relationship. It is important for trainees to learn about these challenges, along with strategies for mitigating them.

One critique of teaching fellows a "mechanistic" approach to working with AYA patients is the concern that it relays a subtext that it is the physician's job to keep these patients engaged in care, minimizing AYA autonomy and agency over their health care. It is important to note, however, that studies of AYA self-management demonstrate that patient-centered communication increases AYA's sense of "relatedness" with their health care providers, and both patient-centered communication and relatedness increased AYA patients' sense of autonomy.[68] Therein, the patient-centered, rapport-building communication strategies emphasized in transitional care are likely to enhance rather than negate AYA autonomy and may improve patient engagement and adherence through this construct.

Importantly, although there is clear evidence that AYA patient outcomes worsen during the time of transition in multiple chronic diseases,[69] and although there is clear evidence that education in transition is currently lacking,[7] with providers in rheumatology[8] and other fields[70-72] feeling unprepared to care for AYA patients, best practice guidelines are largely based on expert opinion, and there is no literature to date demonstrating the link between transition education and improved patient outcomes. This remains a critical need in transition education, within rheumatology and beyond.

Rheumatology has made significant progress in promoting quality transitional care through the development of consensus recommendations for working with young adults,[4-6] and transition tools have been culled and adapted for rheumatologists.[33] However, much remains to be done. Specifically, we must adopt quality improvement and implementation methodology: Plan-Do-Study-Act, whereby "Do" and "Act" entail teaching and role modeling effective care of the AYA patient. When we are able to plan, teach, study, and enhance transitional care best practices, we will be able to train the next generation of rheumatologists to effectively care for an ever-growing population of AYA rheumatology patients.

REFERENCES

1. Jensen PT, Karnes J, Jones K, et al. Quantitative evaluation of a pediatric rheumatology transition program. Pediatr Rheumatol Online J 2015;13:17.
2. Hazel E, Zhang X, Duffy CM, et al. High rates of unsuccessful transfer to adult care among young adults with juvenile idiopathic arthritis. Pediatr Rheumatol Online J 2010;8:2.
3. Hersh A, von Scheven E, Yelin E. Adult outcomes of childhood-onset rheumatic diseases. Nat Rev Rheumatol 2011;7(5):290–5.
4. Foster HE, Minden K, Clemente D, et al. EULAR/PReS standards and recommendations for the transitional care of young people with juvenile-onset rheumatic diseases. Ann Rheum Dis 2017;76(4):639–46.
5. Groot N, de Graeff N, Avcin T, et al. European evidence-based recommendations for diagnosis and treatment of childhood-onset systemic lupus erythematosus: the SHARE initiative. Ann Rheum Dis 2017;76(11):1788–96.
6. Calvo I, Anton J, Bustabad S, et al. Consensus of the Spanish Society of Pediatric Rheumatology for transition management from pediatric to adult care in rheumatic patients with childhood onset. Rheumatol Int 2015;35(10):1615–24.
7. Sadun RE, Chung RJ, Pollock MD, et al. Lost in transition: resident and fellow training and experience caring for young adults with chronic conditions in a large United States' academic medical center. Med Educ Online 2019;24(1):1605783.
8. Zisman D, Samad A, Ardoin SP, et al. US adult rheumatologists' perspective on the transition process for young adults with rheumatic conditions. Arthritis Care Res (Hoboken) 2019. [Epub ahead of print].
9. Brown CR Jr, Criscione-Schreiber L, O'Rourke KS, et al. What is a rheumatologist and how do we make one? Arthritis Care Res (Hoboken) 2016;68(8):1166–72.
10. Available at: http://www.acgme.org/Portals/0/PDFs/Milestones/InternalMedicine SubspecialtyMilestones.pdf. Accessed June 18, 2019.
11. Available at: https://www.rheumatology.org/Portals/0/Files/Adult%20Rheumatology %20EPAs.pdf. Accessed June 18, 2019.
12. Gray WN, Schaefer MR, Resmini-Rawlinson A, et al. Barriers to transition from pediatric to adult care: a systematic review. J Pediatr Psychol 2018;43(5):488–502.
13. Tattersall R, McDonagh JE. Transition: a rheumatology perspective. Br J Hosp Med (Lond) 2010;71(6):315–9.
14. Eleftheriou D, Isenberg DA, Wedderburn LR, et al. The coming of age of adolescent rheumatology. Nat Rev Rheumatol 2014;10(3):187–93.
15. Sadun RE, Schanberg LE. Transition and transfer of the patient with paediatric-onset lupus: a practical approach for paediatric and adult rheumatology practices. Lupus Sci Med 2018;5(1):e000282.
16. Ardoin SP. Transitions in rheumatic disease: pediatric to adult care. Pediatr Clin North Am 2018;65(4):867–83.
17. Chung WW, Hudziak JJ. The transitional age brain: "The Best of Times and the Worst of Times. Child Adolesc Psychiatr Clin N Am 2017;26(2):157–75.

18. Lebel C, Beaulieu C. Longitudinal development of human brain wiring continues from childhood into adulthood. J Neurosci 2011;31(30):10937–47.

19. Colver A, Longwell S. New understanding of adolescent brain development: relevance to transitional healthcare for young people with long term conditions. Arch Dis Child 2013;98(11):902–7.

20. Feldman CH, Collins J, Zhang Z, et al. Dynamic patterns and predictors of hydroxychloroquine nonadherence among Medicaid beneficiaries with systemic lupus erythematosus. Semin Arthritis Rheum 2018;48(2):205–13.

21. Osterberg L, Blaschke T. Adherence to medication. N Engl J Med 2005;353(5): 487–97.

22. Ferro MA, Gorter JW, Boyle MH. Trajectories of depressive symptoms in Canadian emerging adults. Am J Public Health 2015;105(11):2322–7.

23. Ferro MA, Gorter JW, Boyle MH. Trajectories of depressive symptoms during the transition to young adulthood: the role of chronic illness. J Affect Disord 2015;174: 594–601.

24. Thapar A, Collishaw S, Pine DS, et al. Depression in adolescence. Lancet 2012; 379(9820):1056–67.

25. Yu J, Putnick DL, Hendricks C, et al. Health-risk behavior profiles and reciprocal relations with depressive symptoms from adolescence to young adulthood. J Adolesc Health 2017;61(6):773–8.

26. Kann L, McManus T, Harris WA, et al. Youth risk behavior surveillance–United States, 2015. MMWR Surveill Summ 2016;65(6):1–174.

27. Available at: http://www.pewresearch.org/fact-tank/2017/02/13/americans-are-moving-at-historically-low-rates-in-part-because-millennials-are-staying-put/ft_17-02-07_millennial-mobility_2/. Accessed March 8, 2019.

28. Hoeve M, Stams GJ, van der Zouwen M, et al. A systematic review of financial debt in adolescents and young adults: prevalence, correlates and associations with crime. PLoS One 2014;9(8):e104909.

29. Available at: https://www.gottransition.org/resourceGet.cfm?id=5. Accesssed June 24, 2019.

30. Goldenring JM, Cohen E. Getting into adolescent heads. Contemp Pediatr 1988; 5(7):75.

31. Chira P, Ronis T, Ardoin S, et al. Transitioning youth with rheumatic conditions: perspectives of pediatric rheumatology providers in the United States and Canada. J Rheumatol 2014;41(4):768–79.

32. Clemente D, Leon L, Foster H, et al. Transitional care for rheumatic conditions in Europe: current clinical practice and available resources. Pediatr Rheumatol Online J 2017;15(1):49.

33. Available at: https://www.rheumatology.org/Practice-Quality/Pediatric-to-Adult-Rheumatology-Care-Transition. Accessed March 7, 2019.

34. Johnson K, Edens C, Chira P, et al. Differences in healthcare transition views, practices, and barriers among North American Pediatric Rheumatology providers from 2010 to 2018. Arthritis & Rheumatology; 2018. p. 70.

35. Available at: https://www.gottransition.org/about/index.cfm. Accessed March 7, 2019.

36. Available at: https://www.gottransition.org/providers/index.cfm la. Accessed March 7, 2019.

37. Sabbagh S, Ronis T, White PH. Pediatric rheumatology: addressing the transition to adult-orientated health care. Open Access Rheumatol 2018;10:83–95.

38. Hart LC, Pollock M, Brown A, et al. Where Did They Go? Tracking Young Adult Follow-up During the Transition From Pediatric to Adult-Oriented Care. Clin Pediatr (Phila) 2019;58(11-12):1277–83. https://doi.org/10.1177/0009922819852980.

39. Prior M, McManus M, White P, et al. Measuring the "triple aim" in transition care: a systematic review. Pediatrics 2014;134(6):e1648–61.

40. White PH, Cooley WC, Transitions Clinical Report Authoring Group, American Academy of Pediatrics, American Academy of Family Physicians, American College of Physicians. Supporting the Health Care Transition From Adolescence to Adulthood in the Medical Home. Pediatrics 2018;142(5) [pii:e20182587].

41. American Academy of Pediatrics, American Academy of Family Physicians, American College of Physicians, Transitions Clinical Report Authoring Group, Cooley WC, Sagerman PJ. Supporting the health care transition from adolescence to adulthood in the medical home. Pediatrics 2011;128(1):182–200.

42. Coles MS, Greenberg KB. The time is here: a comprehensive curriculum for adolescent health teaching and learning from the Society for Adolescent Health and Medicine. J Adolesc Health 2017;61(2):129–30.

43. Available at: https://www.adolescenthealth.org/Training-and-CME/Adolescent-Medicine-Resident-Curriculum/Adolescent-Medicine-Resident-Curriculum-(9).aspx. Accessed June 24, 2019.

44. Available at: htpps://icaap.remote-learner.net/course/index.php. Accessed June 24, 2019.

45. Fishman L. But Tommy likes it here: moving to adult medicine. MedEdPORTAL 2012;8:9190.

46. Hess JS, Straub DM, Mateus JS, et al. Preparing for transition from pediatric to adult care: evaluation of a physician training program. Adv Pediatr 2015;62(1):137–64.

47. Chung RJ, Jasien J, Maslow GR. Resident dyads providing transition care to adolescents and young adults with chronic illnesses and neurodevelopmental disabilities. J Grad Med Educ 2017;9(2):222–7.

48. Sharma N, O'Hare K, O'Connor KG, et al. Care coordination and comprehensive electronic health records are associated with increased transition planning activities. Acad Pediatr 2018;18(1):111–8.

49. Kuo AA, Ciccarelli MR, Sharma N, et al. A health care transition curriculum for primary care residents: identifying goals and objectives. Pediatrics 2018;141(Suppl 4):S346–54.

50. Sadun R, Maslow G, Chung R, et al. Training adult rheumatology fellows in young adult transition and transfer skills. Arthritis Rheumatol 2017;69. Available at. https://acrabstracts.org/abstract/training-adult-rheumatology-fellows-in-young-adult-transition-and-transfer-skills/.

51. Rosen DS, Blum RW, Britto M, et al. Transition to adult health care for adolescents and young adults with chronic conditions–position paper of the Society for Adolescent Medicine. J Adolesc Health 2003;33(4):309–11.

52. Son MB, Sergeyenko Y, Guan H, et al. Disease activity and transition outcomes in a childhood-onset systemic lupus erythematosus cohort. Lupus 2016;25(13):1431–9.

53. Reiss JG, Gibson RW, Walker LR. Health care transition: youth, family, and provider perspectives. Pediatrics 2005;115(1):112–20.

54. Zhang LF, Ho JS, Kennedy SE. A systematic review of the psychometric properties of transition readiness assessment tools in adolescents with chronic disease. BMC Pediatr 2014;14:4.

55. Sawicki GS, Lukens-Bull K, Yin X, et al. Measuring the transition readiness of youth with special healthcare needs: validation of the TRAQ–Transition Readiness Assessment Questionnaire. J Pediatr Psychol 2011;36(2):160–71.

56. Wood DL, Sawicki GS, Miller MD, et al. The Transition Readiness Assessment Questionnaire (TRAQ): its factor structure, reliability, and validity. Acad Pediatr 2014;14(4):415–22.

57. Jensen PT, Paul GV, LaCount S, et al. Assessment of transition readiness in adolescents and young adults with chronic health conditions. Pediatr Rheumatol Online J 2017;15(1):70.

58. McClellan, C. Trends in Insurance Coverage and Treatment Utilization by Young Adults. The CBHSQ Report: January 29, 2015. Substance Abuse and Mental Health Services Administration, Center for Behavioral Health Statistics and Quality. Rockville, MD. Available at: https://www.ncbi.nlm.nih.gov/books/NBK343536/

59. Carr-Greg M. How to screen an adolescent at risk–HEADSS: the "Review of Systems" for adolescents. Aust J Psychol 2005;57:190.

60. Ford C, English A, Sigman G. Confidential health care for adolescents: position paper for the society for adolescent medicine. J Adolesc Health 2004;35(2):160–7.

61. Sadun RE, Ardoin SP, White PH. Workshop: working with millennials in your practice: skills, tools, and pearls. American College of Rheumatology Annual Meeting; 2018.

62. Mennito S. Resident preferences for a curriculum in healthcare transitions for young adults. South Med J 2012;105(9):462–6.

63. Kolb DA. The process of experiential learning: experience as the source of learning and development. In: Experiential learning. Englewood Cliffs (NJ): Prentice Hall; 1984. p. 20–38. Available at: https://nsee.memberclicks.net/assets/docs/KnowledgeCenter/BuildingExpEduc/BooksReports/27.%20experiential%20learning%20learning%20as%20the%20source.pdf.

64. Knowles M. What is andragogy. In: The modern practice of adult education: from pedagogy to andragogy. Englewood Cliffs (NJ): Prentice Hall; 1980. p. 40–59. Available at: http://www.sciepub.com/reference/131641.

65. Mezirow J. Transformative dimensions of adult learning. San Francisco (CA): Jossey-Bass; 1991.

66. Volertas SD, Rossi-Foulkes R. Using quality improvement in resident education to improve transition care. Pediatr Ann 2017;46(5):e203–6.

67. Peter NG, Forke CM, Ginsburg KR, et al. Transition from pediatric to adult care: internists' perspectives. Pediatrics 2009;123(2):417–23.

68. Johnson KR, McMorris BJ, MapelLentz S, et al. Improving self-management skills through patient-centered communication. J Adolesc Health 2015;57(6):666–72.

69. Betz CL. Approaches to transition in other chronic illnesses and conditions. Pediatr Clin North Am 2010;57(4):983–96.

70. Freed GL, Research Advisory Committee of the American Board of Pediatrics. Comparing perceptions of training for medicine-pediatrics and categorically trained physicians. Pediatrics 2006;118(3):1104–8.

71. Hunt S, Sharma N. Pediatric to adult-care transitions in childhood-onset chronic disease: hospitalist perspectives. J Hosp Med 2013;8(11):627–30.

72. Okumura MJ, Heisler M, Davis MM, et al. Comfort of general internists and general pediatricians in providing care for young adults with chronic illnesses of childhood. J Gen Intern Med 2008;23(10):1621–7.

Ethics and Industry Interactions
Impact on Specialty Training, Clinical Practice, and Research

Jane S. Kang, MD, MS

KEYWORDS

- Ethics • Industry • Rheumatology • Education • Training • Clinical practice
- Research • Trainee

KEY POINTS

- Despite increased awareness of ethical concerns related to industry interactions, there remains a need for interventions to ideally prevent ethical transgressions.
- Mentors perceived to have conflicts of interest or to be engaging in misconduct can unconsciously and profoundly affect the environment by implying certain values and expectations.
- Trainees require tools to organize their thoughts within a bioethical framework to have a systematic, focused, and informed way of approaching ethical issues pertaining to industry interactions.
- Ethics education is essential, but it is likely inadequate in preventing ethical transgressions. Education should be supplemented with ethical environments at local institutions.
- Fears of industry bias should not prevent helpful clinical interactions or innovative research that can help patients. However, integrity is of the utmost importance to maintain the public's trust.

INTRODUCTION

With the growing number of new therapies for rheumatologic diseases, an increased proportion of clinical research in rheumatology is industry funded. Pharmaceutical companies have financial interests, raising a variety of ethical issues in clinical care and research (**Box 1**).

Disclosure Statement: Funding for my project "An Interactive, Case Based, Online Ethics Curriculum for Rheumatology Fellows: Issues in Industry Interactions and Industry Funded Trials" is provided by the Rheumatology Research Foundation Clinician Scholar Educator Award.
Division of Rheumatology, Columbia University Medical Center, 630 West 168th Street, P&S 3-450, New York, NY 10032, USA
E-mail address: jsk2182@columbia.edu

> **Box 1**
> **Ethical considerations for industry interactions in clinical practice and research**
>
> Clinical Practice
> - Gifts, direct financial inducements
> - Drug samples
> - Interactions with pharmaceutical representatives
> - Lectures and presentations
> - Educational resources for physicians
>
> Research
> - Honorary or ghost authorship
> - Financial ties of authors
> - Inadequate and inaccurate disclosures
> - Trial design
> - Data interpretation
> - Composition of manuscript for publication

Physician–pharmaceutical industry relationships are a significant concern of American College of Rheumatology (ACR) members. Although rheumatologists recognize the ethical dilemmas in industry interactions, a survey of the ACR membership found that only 58% of respondents had formal training in ethics and 47% reported having insufficient resources to help them comprehend and resolve ethical matters.[1]

It is important to start discussing these ethical issues with fellows who are likely the most impressionable. Rheumatology fellows need ethics education to prepare them for industry interactions after fellowship. This training is crucial not only for fellows interested in a research career, but also for those planning to be in clinical practice where they may interact with pharmaceutical representatives, recruit patients for industry-funded trials, or interpret data from industry-funded trials.

The Accreditation Council for Graduate Medical Education (ACGME) requires rheumatology faculty and fellows to adhere to ethical principles. Additionally, the ACGME gives guidelines pertaining to research ethics, stating that fellows must demonstrate knowledge of "the essential components of quality experimental design, clinical trial design, data analysis, and interpretation of results, and the importance of adherence to ethical standards of experimentation."[2]

Some may argue that additional training in ethics is redundant for rheumatology fellows, because many of them take online courses that their institutions require, such as the Collaborative Institutional Training Initiative (CITI) program online. However, existing programs are very general, may superficially address key issues, and are not specific to rheumatology. One can pass the modules by skipping the required reading and answering the mandatory questions at the end.

Because rheumatologists do not feel they have the knowledge or tools to assess bioethical matters they encounter,[1] improving knowledge of bioethics and applying that knowledge to assess ethical issues is essential. We should give our trainees the tools to organize their thoughts within a bioethical framework, so that they have a systematic, focused, and informed way of approaching ethical issues pertaining to industry interactions and industry-funded clinical research.

ACADEMIA AND INDUSTRY

Enactment of the Bayh-Dole Act or the Patent and Trademark Law Amendments Act in 1980[3] encouraged the transfer of new advancements from the university to the private sector, increasing university patent licensing. Subsequently, a new model for revenue at academic institutions was introduced, increasing entrepreneurialism by medical centers. Industry financing has also increased, further obscuring the boundaries between academic and commercial principles.

The growing research collaborations between academia and pharmaceutical, medical device, and biotechnology companies has raised concerns regarding COI, potentially causing undue influence. In 2007, the Institute of Medicine elected the Committee on Conflict of Interest in Medical Research, Education, and Practice to examine these issues, and issued a report that emphasizes preventive measures to avoid bias and mistrust that threatens the integrity of researchers, objectivity of medical education, quality of patient care and the public's trust in medicine.[4]

Concerns with industry interactions should not prevent relationships that can help patients. Although trainees are largely protected from industry, the reality is that after their undergraduate and graduate medical training, they will frequently encounter industry interactions. It is our duty as educators to prepare our rheumatology fellows for that reality.

ETHICAL CONSIDERATIONS FOR INDUSTRY INTERACTIONS IN CLINICAL PRACTICE

In 2007, a study found that most physicians (94%) reported some type of relationship with industry, most of them relating to receiving food at work (83%) or receiving drug samples (78%).[5] With the advent of the Physician Payments Sunshine Act, a physician's financial ties to industry are now publicly reported.[6]

Although trainees are generally protected from industry interactions in the academic setting, they still have some exposure to industry and receive offers for industry-sponsored gifts. In 2013, a national survey of third- and fourth-year medical students and third-year residents found that offers for industry-sponsored gifts are common (33% of first-year students, 57% of fourth-year students, and 54% of residents), which includes meals outside of the hospital and free drug samples.[7]

We know that gifts or other direct financial inducements from industry can affect prescribing behavior of physicians. Social science research shows that even small gifts may influence physicians and lead to a COI.[8] In radiation oncology, those who accepted larger gifts were far more likely to disagree with regulations that would discourage gift giving.[9]

Free drug samples can also affect physician prescribing behavior. Clinicians who had samples in their office were more likely to prescribe drugs that were different from their preferred drug choice[10] and less likely to prescribe first-line, preferred medications.[11]

Trainees' prescribing behavior can also be influenced by interactions with pharmaceutical representatives.[12] Residents who had access to drug samples were less likely to initiate therapy with unadvertised drugs than residents who did not have access to drug samples.[13] In a study evaluating self-reported prescribing patterns for 3 clinical scenarios (uncomplicated urinary tract infection, hypertension, and depression), residents and younger physicians were more likely to use drug samples in 2 or more of these scenarios compared with attendings.[10]

The type of clinical experiences trainees have had can affect their likelihood of exposure to pharmaceutical marketing. Medical students at rural sites reported more exposure to pharmaceutical marketing than in urban sites. Compared with urban sites, physicians meeting with pharmaceutical representatives were 4 times higher in rural sites (40% vs 10%) and distribution of drug samples was 3 times higher in rural sites (54% vs 15%).[14]

More internal medicine residents than faculty believed that income or gifts from industry influences teaching in different educational contexts, including rounds, in-hospital lectures and journal clubs, and out-of-hospital dinner lectures and journal clubs. Most internal medicine residents and faculty perceived that income or gifts from industry influences how visiting attendings teach in-hospital lectures such as grand rounds and out-of-hospital dinner lectures and journal clubs.[15]

At 1 university hospital, residents who attended grand rounds given by a pharmaceutical employee were surveyed after 3 months; those who attended the grand rounds were more likely to choose the drug made by the speaker's company, which was more expensive, even if it was not the best choice.[16]

Pharmaceutical representatives may offer educational materials to trainees. Although medical students are unlikely to remember the specific pharmaceutical companies that gave them a free textbook, their interactions with pharmaceutical representatives were likely to be viewed as "helpful and informative."[17]

The perception that industry interactions lead to bias is prevalent among trainees, but the belief that these interactions provide valuable education for physicians increases over the course of undergraduate and graduate medical education (64% of first-year students, 68% of fourth-year students, 80% of residents).[7] Clinical students were more likely than preclinical students to state that promotional information is helpful for learning about new medications. Additionally, the frequency of contact is correlated with favorable attitudes toward industry interactions.[18]

Students at medical schools with more restrictive policies regarding pharmaceutical company interactions were less likely to accept gifts and interact with pharmaceutical representatives.[7,19] However, there is evidence that these behavioral effects of restrictive policies in medical school do not persist into residency,[20] suggesting that consistency and rigor of policies in graduate medical education is just as important.

EDUCATIONAL INTERVENTIONS FOR INDUSTRY INTERACTIONS IN CLINICAL PRACTICE

The existence of ethics codes alone is not sufficient to prevent physicians from ethical transgressions. It is vital to discuss ethical issues related to industry interactions as early as possible in medical training, and it should continue throughout and after training. Trainees should receive education on COI that includes both didactics and case-based discussions on topics including disclosing commercial interests, avoiding actual or perceived COI, and managing industry interactions.[21]

In a study involving focus groups, physicians appreciated the value of transparency, but did not view the Physician Payments Sunshine Act (PPSA) as helping increase scientific integrity or patient trust. Rather, physicians felt that the PPSA was a threat to their privacy and reputation.[22]

Making people aware of their potential biases does not seem to decrease these biases significantly. This bias blind spot makes us feel more assured of our own judgments and more critical of other's biases.[23]

There are also substantial gaps and variations in understanding COI. Many physicians are skeptical of the existing evidence showing that industry can influence practice decisions.[22] Internal medicine residents and faculty have reported low levels of knowledge regarding physician–pharmaceutical industry interactions.[24] Therefore, educating physicians about the basic principles of COI is imperative.

Educational interventions can affect medical students' attitudes about physician interactions with the pharmaceutical industry[25,26] and industry-related behaviors.[26] In a prospective cohort study of a graduating medical student class, the students who received educational interventions regarding pharmaceutical marketing (live presentation, faculty debate, and an interactive Web-based course) were more likely than control students to believe that physicians are influenced by pharmaceutical marketing and more likely to prescribe a company's drug if they received gifts and food from that company. Students who received the educational interventions were also more likely to support banning interactions between pharmaceutical representatives, students, and physicians.[25]

At 1 academic institution, internal medicine residents were followed more than 3 years after being given an interactive educational workshop (reviews of literature and guidelines and 3 videos on resident–industry interactions). The educational workshop resulted in small changes in their perceptions of industry interactions that were in line with the existing residency policies,[27] suggesting that institutional policies are also an important way to reinforce the educational aims of ethics education.

Restricting interactions between pharmaceutical representatives and internal medicine residents can be effective. In a retrospective study analyzing the attitudes and behaviors of physicians, those who trained with restrictive policies regarding industry interactions were less likely to believe that pharmaceutical representative information was beneficial and had less current contact with pharmaceutical representatives. The physicians surveyed were at least 3 years out of residency.[28]

Another proposed model involves a partnership between industry and educators to prepare trainees for industry interactions. One study evaluated the effects of a workshop for third-year medical students facilitated by 2 faculty members and a regional manager of pharmaceutical representatives from a major pharmaceutical company. After the workshop, the perceived educational value of pharmaceutical representative information to practicing physicians and medical students was higher (18% to 43%) and the perceived degree of bias of pharmaceutical representative information decreased (84% to 73%), but the perceived degree of influence on prescribing increased (44% to 62%).[29]

A key question is how many graduate medical programs have educational interventions to address industry interactions. A survey of United States family medicine program directors revealed that less than one-half of US family medicine programs have a curriculum that addresses physician–industry interactions. A formal curriculum was more likely in residencies that allowed industry interactions or were affiliated with a university.[30]

The more restrictive approach to industry interactions in graduate medical education may be the reason why programs deem a formal curriculum unnecessary. Between 2008 and 2013, industry interactions have decreased in family medicine programs. Family medicine programs not accepting gifts or meals from industry increased from 48% to 73%, refusing samples increased from 52% to 78%, and restricting access to residents increased from 43% to 74%. However, industry-sponsored activities stayed the same (67% to 73%).[31]

Perhaps there is increased awareness of industry-related ethical considerations among trainees. At 1 medical school, students were more aware of the potential affects of industry interactions[32] compared with prior studies.[33]

ETHICAL CONSIDERATIONS FOR INDUSTRY-FUNDED RESEARCH

There has been an enormous growth of therapies available for rheumatologic diseases, resulting in an increased proportion of clinical research in rheumatology being sponsored by industry. Pharmaceutical companies have financial interests and can play a large part in study design, data interpretation, and the composition of a manuscript for publication.

Honorary or ghost authorship by academic faculty of industry-sponsored trials is used to give legitimacy to a trial. In 2008, the prevalence of honorary and ghost authors in 6 high-impact medical journals was 21%, compared to 29.2% in 1996.[34] The persistently high prevalence of honorary and ghost authors suggests the need to increase efforts to promote scientific integrity.

A survey of lead academic authors found that in the majority of industry-funded trials published in high-impact journals, the industry funder influenced all components of the trials. Also, these academic authors noted that access to the data did not mean they would always have complete access, and data analysis was often done without academic involvement. Although lead academic authors found industry collaborations beneficial, some described a decrease in academic freedom, such as delays in publication by the industry funder and disagreements on trial design and reporting with the industry funder.[35]

Trials funded by industry or for-profit organizations can result in biased findings.[36–40] Studies sponsored only by for-profit organizations were significantly more likely to favor the experimental treatment compared with studies without financial competing interests (ie, financial gain or loss depending on outcomes) or trials funded by both for-profit and nonprofit organizations.[38]

In a study investigating 103 randomized controlled trials (RCTs) for rheumatoid arthritis (RA), 56.3% were funded by industry, 18.4% by nonprofit sources, and 5.8% had mixed funding. However, the source of funding was not associated with positive results for the industry sponsored drug. A trend toward a higher nonpublication rate of industry-funded trials was observed, perhaps indicating that publication bias is partially responsible for this lack of association.[41]

Contradictory findings were noted in a study evaluating abstracts presented at the 2001 ACR annual meeting. The maintenance of clinical equipoise in industry-sponsored rheumatologic studies was reviewed in abstracts of RCTs accepted for the 2001 ACR annual meeting. Of the 45 trials studied, all 45 studies favored the sponsor's drug.[42] Design bias, which involves using extensive preliminary data to design studies that will have a higher likelihood of favoring the sponsor's drug, may have contributed to positive findings in all the industry-sponsored trials.

It is critical to consider not only funding source, but also financial ties of the individual authors. In a review of RCTs published in core clinical journals in 2013, financial ties of the principle investigators were independently associated with a positive result.[43] Among authors of RCTs for RA, potential financial COI is common and increasing. An author's receipt of honoraria or consulting fees increased the likelihood of a positive RA study outcome.[44]

Financial COI has also been assessed in fibromyalgia drug therapy RCTs, most of which are industry sponsored. After adjusting for sample size, there was no association between industry funding or authors' financial COI (honoraria or consulting fees) and study outcome.[45]

Despite an increased awareness of COI in medicine, physicians are not disclosing all their financial relationships. A study found that 32% of oncology authors did not fully disclose industry payments from oncology drug clinical trials published in major medical journals.[46] This finding supports other studies that have found that COI disclosures in medical journals are inadequate.[4,39,47]

COI disclosures are available for RCTs, but less commonly for meta-analyses. When considering published studies in high-impact medical journals for patented pharmacotherapies across various medicine subspecialties, information about the study funding and author COI for the RCTs included in the meta-analysis were seldom reported.[48]

Industry's increasing presence in clinical trials has implications for clinical practice guidelines and how we interpret them. Recent studies have found incomplete or inaccurate disclosures of authors of dermatology[49] and otolaryngology clinical practice guidelines.[50] The ACR guideline development process has evolved to ensure integrity,[51] and yet financial COI in ACR clinical guidelines have also been critiqued.[52]

In thinking about COI, we must consider the accuracy of public data, relevance of the financial ties to the guidelines being considered, and the monetary amount. Nonfinancial COI, such as intellectual conflicts, are difficult to capture or measure, but also raise concerns.

There are social science concepts to consider as well, such as self-serving bias, strategic exaggeration, and moral licensing. With self-serving bias, the physician considering pharmaceutical research data may unknowingly look at equivocal or weak data in favor of a product.[8,23] Strategic exaggeration is the tendency to provide more biased recommendations to counteract the expected discounting of the recommendations. Moral licensing is the unconscious sentiment that biased recommendations are acceptable because disclosures were given.[53]

Complete and accurate disclosures may help readers interpret results appropriately and consider potential biases. However, the effects of disclosure are mixed. Sometimes disclosure of financial connections can be seen as a measure of expertise.[54] Conversely, declaring a COI does not necessarily erase the negative perceptions or biases in industry-funded research.[55]

Physicians diminish the credibility of research when the authors are employees of a company that can benefit from the study, but did not do so when the authors are not employees of the company but received grants from the company.[56,57] Although physicians may feel that they should devalue information from conflicted sources, they actually may not do so until they are given a direct comparison between 2 studies with and without conflicts.[58]

Compared with trials in which no disclosure statement was included, physicians were less likely to see industry trials as having a high level of rigor and less likely to have confidence in the results. Even when study methods were the same between industry-funded and non–industry-funded trials, physicians felt that the industry-funded studies were not as rigorously conducted. Compared with trials funded by the National Institutes of Health (NIH), physicians were also less likely to consider industry trials as important and less likely to prescribe the drugs being investigated by industry.[59]

However, the quality of trials seems to be equivalent between industry and non-industry,[37,38,40] and this finding is also the case in rheumatologic trials.[60] Specifically, industry-funded trials for RA have been shown to be equivalent to non–industry-funded trials.[61] However, the RA trials evaluated were those done in 1989 or earlier, which is before the use of tumor necrosis factor inhibitors and other biologics in clinical practice. Additionally, assessing factors such as randomization and blinding are not sufficient to evaluate trial quality.

Other factors such as the use of appropriate control therapies must also be taken into account. The use of placebo is favored in industry trials,[37,38] including those for RA.[62] Avoiding the use of inactive controls does not eliminate the potential for bias: the comparator drug may be used in lower doses.[36] This phenomenon of subtherapeutic dosing has also been noted with methotrexate and allopurinol dosing in RA[63] and gout trials.[64]

Many pharmaceutical companies prefer to conduct research in foreign (especially developing) countries because of the cost savings.[65] In fact, rheumatology research abroad in developing countries, such as the Asia-Pacific region,[66] is increasingly prevalent. Numerous factors such as poverty, illiteracy, cultural influences, lack of or inadequate access to health care, and substandard research infrastructures, all make recruitment in developing countries ethically complicated, and may take advantage of a vulnerable population. Conducting studies abroad, especially in developing countries, can allow greater access to a larger population that have not been on treatment, either due to access issues or differences in treatment of a disease between countries. Study participants abroad may not have access to what is considered standard of care in the United States.

EDUCATIONAL INTERVENTIONS FOR INDUSTRY-FUNDED RESEARCH

Federal mandates require instruction in research integrity for all federally funded research trainees. The US Office of Research Integrity promotes responsible conduct of research (RCR), assuming this will be vital in encouraging ethical behavior.

One research ethics course early in a young researcher's career is not enough to result in long-term retention of knowledge.[67] Trainees should be exposed to research ethics training more than once, because their experiences broaden over time, with questions and issues becoming more intricate and challenging.[68] Research ethics education should start early and continue throughout all levels of medical training.

Trainees overall evaluate research ethics training, such as RCR courses, positively. They feel that these courses help them acquire knowledge about research misconduct and learn how to avoid and respond to it. Ethics teaching has also been associated with increased appropriate answers to questions related to publication and authorship.[69] However, RCR courses may more greatly influence knowledge than changes in skills or attitudes.[69,70]

Trainees with limited RCR exposure or who agreed with what was being taught are more readily influenced and perhaps more likely to integrate new information in future ethical dilemmas. Those with prior experiences or existing knowledge that diverged from what was being taught often challenged or rejected the new ideas that were being discussed,[68] supporting the argument that research ethics education should begin early, before beliefs are consolidated and difficult to change.

In a survey of researchers, a high proportion of them did not receive dedicated training in research ethics. Early career researchers with funding from the NIH who had received research ethics training were more likely to engage in questionable research behaviors related to their study data than those without such training.[71] This finding may be a result of the educational intervention being given too late, after ideas and opinions are solidified. Others have found that reported ethics training was not associated with a difference in past[72] or potential research misbehaviors.[72,73]

Mentoring has varied effects on ethical transgressions in research.[71] Mentees may ultimately do what their mentors want because it is difficult for them to disagree. A mentor–mentee system and role modeling are important, but likely not sufficient to prevent unethical behavior in clinical research.

In research, a major factor to consider is trainees observing attending behavior in industry interactions, and the unintended and vast effects attending behaviors can have in implying certain values and expectations in the learning environment.

THE HIDDEN CURRICULUM IN RESEARCH

If trainees learn professional and ethical standards through their research mentors, the mentors must be aware of ethical standards and behave ethically. Faculty are often unclear about what is considered ethical[74] and can be involved in unethical research practices themselves.[75,76] One study found that only 50% of university health education faculty received formal teaching in research and publishing ethics at the universities in which they work.[74] The variation in what is considered ethical and the lack of formal research ethics teaching is problematic.

Although major cases of scientific misconduct revolve around falsification, fabrication, and plagiarism, scientists more commonly engage in other questionable behaviors that cross the ethical line in research.[75] These regular or normal misbehaviors (such as changing the design, methodology, or results of a study in response to pressure from a funding source or publishing the same data or results in 2 or more publications) may be more of a threat to the integrity of research rather than the attention-grabbing, notorious cases involving falsification, fabrication, and plagiarism.[76]

Midcareer researchers are more likely to engage in research misconduct compared with early career researchers (38% and 28%, respectively).[76] Perhaps early career researchers were more afraid to report transgressions. Another possibility is that midcareer researchers learn to misbehave over time, owing to observation, experience, or opportunities to misbehave where they received their training and where they work currently.

Trainees not only observe misconduct, but also can be involved in misconduct themselves, and may be more likely to be involved in unethical behavior if they have witnessed misconduct. In highly competitive departments, where students have to compete for resources and faculty attention, graduate students are significantly more likely to observe research misconduct by peers and faculty.[77]

These findings are especially concerning because faculty serve as role models for students, trainees, and younger professionals. If faculty are perceived to be engaging in research misconduct, they can have unconscious and profound effects on the learning and academic environment by implying certain values and expectations. Varying opinions on what is considered ethical has implications for reprimanding those who behave unethically and preventing research misbehavior.

Responsible investigators who observe research misconduct may fear reporting the irresponsibility of others. In a survey of medical school based researchers who were principal investigators on grants from the NIH, those who correctly identified instances of research misconduct were extremely unlikely to report it to a research integrity officer.[78] Improving the quality of mentoring at training programs and protecting whistleblowers is crucial.

AN INTERACTIVE, CASE-BASED, ONLINE ETHICS CURRICULUM

We should not only be concerned if ethical considerations related to industry interactions are being taught, but also (1) who is being taught, (2) how it is being taught, and (3) if it can improve knowledge or behavior. There is evidence to show that appropriate teaching methods could affect moral reasoning: small group discussions of case studies may be more effective in developing moral reasoning compared with lectures.[79]

Bioethics education usually includes lectures and small group discussions, but computerized learning may be just as, or more, effective. At 1 medical school, one-half of a medical student class received bioethics lectures and small group discussions, and the other half received a similar course, except that 2 group discussions were replaced with a computer-based learning program. Although the examination scores were comparable between the 2 groups, the students who received the computer-based learning program scored higher in certain examination areas and evaluated the course slightly better.[80]

Regarding ethics education, the ACR membership also prefers web-based programs compared with in-person sessions and journal articles.[1] There are both advantages and disadvantages of using computer based learning modules. It is worth highlighting the advantages[80]:

- Self-paced learning
- Simulation of real-world cases
- Feedback provided in real time
- Ability to record answers anonymously
- Consistency of the learning material
- Avoidance of small group variability
- Avoidance of peer pressure influence

Since 2012, I have been teaching our rheumatology fellows key ethical concerns through interactive small group activities and case-based discussions that cover the history and principles of bioethics and codes and regulations pertinent to clinical and research ethics. Fellows also perform a bioethical analysis of their second year research projects; I have created a detailed guide to help fellows deeply consider each of the bioethical principles and how they may apply to their own research projects.

Despite required, standardized institutional training (such as the CITI program), I have realized that the fellows need to improve their knowledge of the basic principles of bioethics, therefore lacking an appropriate framework to systematically analyze ethical issues. Currently, I am expanding their ethics education into a more extensive curriculum using interactive, case-based, online modules with the goal of improving the fellows' knowledge of bioethical principles and ability to assess bioethical issues in industry interactions and research. Online modules also allow for easier portability of the curriculum for dissemination to other rheumatology fellowships, which can then be completed in the fellows' own time (and repeated if desired) or during dedicated time established by fellowship programs.

The online curriculum starts with knowledge acquisition (history, principles, codes, and regulations), with later modules requiring fellows to recall and apply bioethical principles to analyze and evaluate industry interactions in clinical practice, industry-funded rheumatology clinical research, and their own clinical cases and research projects. Knowledge retention is promoted by activating prior and new knowledge when working through simulated cases with real world applications to develop their critical thinking skills in ethics.

ENSURING ETHICAL INDUSTRY INTERACTIONS IN RHEUMATOLOGY

Integrity is of the utmost importance in medicine to maintain the public's trust in physicians and the research enterprise. On an institutional level, self-regulation is indispensable. Academic centers must not only protect whistleblowers, but also cultivate an environment where possible ethical transgressions can be discussed without fear.

Ideally, ethical transgressions should be prevented. Primary prevention, or preventing unethical behavior by identifying and removing causal factors, is the most appealing intervention. However, secondary prevention to prevent someone who has engaged in minor ethical misbehaviors from engaging in more serious transgressions is also a major consideration.

Codes and regulations are necessary, but ultimately we must nurture trainees to become ethically conscientious physicians. We should not minimize the value of educational interventions early on in training to ensure ethical interactions with industry. Young physicians in training must be cognizant of ethical concerns related to industry and learn to use bioethical principles when faced with ethical dilemmas in clinical care and research. Continued learning is essential, even as trainees move on to faculty positions, where they will serve as mentors.

We must also educate mentors in rheumatology, who serve as role models for trainees. Academic rheumatologists may be the ones with the most influence in clinical care and research, and therefore would be able to reform particular paradigms of structural ethical negligence. Ethics education or mentoring alone is likely insufficient: both are important and necessary.

Although ethics education may not prevent all types of ethical misbehavior, improving knowledge in this area is an essential step in the right direction. Educating rheumatology faculty and trainees may help transform the way we think about and manage industry interactions and industry-funded research.

Fears of industry bias should not prevent helpful clinical interactions or innovative research that can help patients. However, we must be vigilant about considering potential biases and areas of ethical uncertainties that do not uphold the inviolable trust between the patient and physician, and the integrity of the clinical research enterprise.

ACKNOWLEDGMENTS

The author wishes to thank Robert Klitzman for reviewing this article.

REFERENCES

1. MacKenzie CR, Meltzer M, Kitsis EA, et al. Ethical challenges in rheumatology: a survey of the American College of Rheumatology membership. Arthritis Rheum 2013;65(10):2524–32.
2. ACGME Program Requirements for Graduate Medical Education in Rheumatology. Accreditation Council for Graduate Medical Education. Available at: https://www.acgme.org/Portals/0/PFAssets/ProgramRequirements/150_Rheumatology_2019.pdf?ver=2019-06-21-003544-283. Accessed October 3, 2019.
3. Chapter 18 – Patent Rights in Inventions Made with Federal Assistance. Title 35 – Patents. Available at: http://www.gpo.gov/fdsys/pkg/USCODE-2011-title35/pdf/USCODE-2011-title35-partII-chap18.pdf. Accessed October 3, 2019.
4. Committee on Conflict of Interest in Medical Research, Education, and Practice, Board on Health Sciences Policy. In: Lo B, Field MJ, editors. Conflict of interest in medical research, education, and practice. Washington, DC: National Academies Press; 2009.
5. Campbell EG, Gruen RL, Mountford J, et al. A national survey of physician-industry relationships. N Engl J Med 2007;356:1742–50.
6. Open Payments. Centers for Medicare & Medicaid Services. Available at: http://www.cms.gov/openpayments/. Accessed October 3, 2019.
7. Austad KE, Avorn J, Franklin JM, et al. Changing interactions between physician trainees and the pharmaceutical industry: a national survey. J Gen Intern Med 2013;28(8):1064–71.

8. Dana J, Loewenstein G. A social science perspective on gifts to physicians from industry. JAMA 2003;290:252–5.

9. Halperin EC, Hutchison P, Barrier RC Jr. A population-based study of the prevalence and influence of gifts to radiation oncologists from pharmaceutical companies and medical equipment manufacturers. Int J Radiat Oncol Biol Phys 2004;59(5):1477–83.

10. Chew LD, O'Young TS, Hazlet TK, et al. A physician survey of the effect of drug sample availability on physicians' behavior. J Gen Intern Med 2000;15(7):478–83.

11. Pinckney RG, Helminski AS, Kennedy AG, et al. The effect of medication samples on self-reported prescribing practices: a statewide, cross-sectional survey. J Gen Intern Med 2011;26(1):40–4.

12. Zipkin DA, Steinman MA. Interactions between pharmaceutical representatives and doctors in training a thematic review. J Gen Intern Med 2005;20:777–86.

13. Adair RF, Holmgren LR. So drug samples influence resident prescribing behavior? A randomized trial. Am J Med 2005;118(8):881–4.

14. Evans DV, Keys T, Desnick L, et al. Big pharma on the farm: students are exposed to pharmaceutical marketing more often more often in rural clinics. Fam Med 2016;48(7):561–4.

15. Watson PY, Khandelwal AK, Musial JL, et al. Resident and faculty perceptions of conflict of interest in medical education. J Gen Intern Med 2005;20(4):357–9.

16. Spingarn RW, Berlin JA, Strom BL. When pharmaceutical manufacturers' employees present grand rounds, what do residents remember? Acad Med 1996; 71(1):86–8.

17. Sandberg WS, Carlos R, Sandberg EH, et al. The effect of educational gifts from pharmaceutical firms on medical students' recall of company names or products. Acad Med 1997;72(10):916–8.

18. Austad KE, Avorn J, Kesselheim AS. Medical students' exposure to and attitudes about the pharmaceutical industry: a systematic review. PLoS Med 2011;8(5): e1001037.

19. Yeh JS, Austad KE, Franklin JM, et al. Association of medical students' reports of interactions with the pharmaceutical and medical device industries and medical school policies and characteristics: a cross- sectional study. PLoS Med 2014; 11(10):e1001743.

20. Yeh JS, Austad KE, Franklin JM, et al. Medical schools' industry interaction policies not associated with trainees' self-reported behavior as residents: results of a national survey. J Grad Med Educ 2015;7(4):595–602.

21. Wayne DB, Green M, Neilson EG. Teaching medical students about conflicts of interest. JAMA 2017;317(17):1733–4.

22. Chimonas S, DeVito NJ, Rothman DJ. Bringing transparency to medicine: exploring physicians' views and experiences of the Sunshine Act. Am J Bioeth 2017;17(6):4–18.

23. Dana J. Appendix D: how psychological research can inform policies for dealing with conflict of interest in medicine. In: Lo B, Field MJ, editors. Conflict of interest in medical research, education, and practice. Washington, DC: National Academies Press; 2009. p. 358–74.

24. Watkins R, Kimberly J. What residents don't know about physician-pharmaceutical industry interactions. Acad Med 2004;79(5):432–7.

25. Kao AC, Braddock C, Clay M, et al. Effect of educational interventions and medical school policies on medical students' attitudes toward pharmaceutical marketing practices: a multi-institutional study. Acad Med 2011;86:1454–62.

26. Carroll AE, Vreeman RC, Buddenbaum J, et al. To what extent do educational interventions impact medical trainees' attitudes and behaviors regarding industry-trainee and industry-physician relationships? Pediatrics 2007;120(6):e1528–35.
27. Schneider JA, Arora V, Kasza K, et al. Residents' perceptions over time of pharmaceutical industry interactions and gifts and the effect of an educational intervention. Acad Med 2006;81(7):595–602.
28. McCormick BB, Tomlinson G, Brill-Edwards P, et al. Effect of restricting contact between pharmaceutical company representatives and internal medicine residents on posttraining attitudes and behavior. JAMA 2001;286(16):1994–9.
29. Wofford JL, Ohl CA. Teaching appropriate interactions with pharmaceutical company representatives: the impact of an innovative workshop on student attitudes. BMC Med Educ 2005;5(1):5.
30. Evans DV, Waters RC, Olsen C, et al. Residency curricula on physician-pharmaceutical industry interaction: a CERA study. Fam Med 2016;48(1):44–8.
31. Brown SR, Evans DV, Fugh-Berman A. Pharmaceutical industry interactions in family medicine residencies decreased between 2008 and 2013: a CERA study. Fam Med 2015;47(4):279–82.
32. Kim A, Mumm LA, Korenstein D. Routine conflict of interest disclosure by preclinical lecturers and medical students' attitudes toward the pharmaceutical and device industries. JAMA 2012;308(21):2187–9.
33. Sierles FS, Brodkey AC, Cleary LM, et al. Medical students' exposure to and attitudes about drug company interactions: a national survey. JAMA 2005;294(9):1034–42.
34. Wislar JS, Flanagin A, Fontanarosa PB, et al. Honorary and ghost authorship in high impact biomedical journals: a cross sectional survey. BMJ 2011;343:d6128.
35. Rasmussen K, Bero L, Redberg R, et al. Collaboration between academics and industry in clinical trials: cross sectional study of publications and survey of lead academic authors. BMJ 2018;363:k3654.
36. Rochon PA, Gurwitz JH, Simms RW, et al. A study of manufacturer-supported trials of nonsteroidal anti-inflammatory drugs in the treatment of arthritis. Arch Intern Med 1994;154:157–63.
37. Djulbegovic B, Lacevic M, Cantor A, et al. The uncertainty principle and industry-sponsored research. Lancet 2000;356:635–8.
38. Kjaergard LL, Als-Nielsen B. Association between competing interests and authors' conclusions: epidemiological study of randomised clinical trials published in the BMJ. BMJ 2002;325:249.
39. Bekelman JE, Li Y, Gross CP. Scope and impact of financial conflicts of interest in biomedical research: a systemic review. JAMA 2003;289(4):454–65.
40. Lexchin J, Bero LA, Djulbegovic B, et al. Pharmaceutical industry sponsorship and research outcome and quality: systematic review. BMJ 2003;326:1167–70.
41. Khan NA, Lombeida JI, Singh M, et al. Association of industry funding with the outcome and quality of randomized controlled trials of drug therapy for rheumatoid arthritis. Arthritis Rheum 2012;64(7):2059–67.
42. Fries JF, Equipoise Krishnan E. design bias, and randomized controlled trials: the elusive ethics of new drug development. Arthritis Res Ther 2004;6(3):R250–5.
43. Ahn R, Woodbridge A, Abraham A, et al. Financial ties of principal investigators and randomized controlled trial outcomes: cross sectional study. BMJ 2017;356:i6770.
44. Khan NA, Nguyen CL, Khawar T, et al. Association of author's financial conflict of interest with characteristics and outcome of rheumatoid arthritis randomized

controlled trials. Rheumatology (Oxford) 2018. https://doi.org/10.1093/rheumatology/key368.

45. Pang WK, Yeter KC, Torralba KD, et al. Financial conflicts of interest and their association with outcome and quality of fibromyalgia drug therapy randomized controlled trials. Int J Rheum Dis 2015;18(6):606–15.

46. Wayant C, Turner E, Meyer C, et al. Financial conflicts of interest among oncologist authors of reports of clinical drug trials. JAMA Oncol 2018;4(10):1426–8.

47. Grundy Q, Dunn AG, Bourgeois FT, et al. Prevalence of disclosed conflicts of interest in biomedical research and associations with journal impact factors and altmetric scores. JAMA 2018;319(4):408–9.

48. Roseman M, Milette K, Bero LA, et al. Reporting of conflicts of interest in meta-analyses of trials of pharmacological treatments. JAMA 2011;305(10):1008–17.

49. Checketts JX, Sims MT, Vassar M. Evaluating industry payments among dermatology clinical practice guidelines authors. JAMA Dermatol 2017;153(12):1229–35.

50. Horn J, Checketts JX, Jawhar O, et al. Evaluation of industry relationships among authors of otolaryngology clinical practice guidelines. JAMA Otolaryngol Head Neck Surg 2018;144(3):194–201.

51. Yazdany J, Caplan L, Fitzgerald J, et al. Editorial: the evolving art and science of American College of Rheumatology guidelines. Arthritis Rheumatol 2019;71(1):2–4.

52. Khan R, Scaffidi MA, Rumman A, et al. Prevalence of financial conflicts of interest among authors of clinical guidelines related to high-revenue medications. JAMA Intern Med 2018;178(12):1712–5.

53. Loewenstein G, Sah S, Cain DM. The unintended consequences of conflict of interest disclosure. JAMA 2012;307(7):669–70.

54. Cain DM, Loewenstein G, Moore DA. The dirt on coming clean: possible effects of disclosing conflicts of interest. J Legal Stud 2005;34:1–24.

55. Rosenbaum L. Understanding bias – the case for careful study. N Engl J Med 2015;372(20):1959–63.

56. Chaudhry S, Schroter S, Smith R, et al. Does declaration of competing interest affect readers' perceptions? A randomised trial. BMJ 2002;325:1391–2.

57. Schroter S, Morris J, Chaudry S, et al. Does the type of competing interest statement affect readers' perceptions of the credibility of research? Randomised trial. BMJ 2004;328:742–3.

58. Silverman GK, Loewenstein GF, Anderson BL, et al. Failure to discount for conflict of interest when evaluating medical literature: a randomised trial of physicians. J Med Ethics 2010;36:265–70.

59. Kesselheim AS, Robertson CT, Myers JA, et al. A randomized study of how physicians interpret research funding disclosures. N Engl J Med 2012;367:1119–27.

60. Hill CL, LaValley MP, Felson DT. Secular changes in the quality of published randomized clinical trials in rheumatology. Arthritis Rheum 2002;46:779–84.

61. Anderson JJ, Felson DT, Meenan RF. Secular changes in published clinical trials of second-line agents in rheumatoid arthritis. Arthritis Rheum 1991;34:1304–9.

62. Estellat C, Ravaud P. Lack of head-to-head trials and fair control arms: randomized controlled trials of biologic treatment for rheumatoid arthritis. Arch Intern Med 2012;172(3):237–44.

63. Estellat C, Tubach F, Seror R, et al. Control treatments in biologics trials of rheumatoid arthritis were often not deemed acceptable in the context of care. J Clin Epidemiol 2016;69:235–44.

64. Shmerling RH. Editorial: the ethics of recent gout trials. Arthritis Rheumatol 2016; 68(9):2057–60.
65. Garnier J. Rebuilding the R&D engine in big pharma. Harv Bus Rev 2008;86: 68–76.
66. Torralba KD, Khan NA, Quismorio FP. Clinical trials and public trust: the geographical shift to the Asia-Pacific region. Int J Rheum Dis 2009;12:186–91.
67. Heitman E, Olsen CH, Anestidou L, et al. New graduate students' baseline knowledge of the responsible conduct of research. Acad Med 2007;82:838–45.
68. Mcgee R, Almquist J, Keller JL, et al. Teaching and learning responsible research conduct: influences of prior experiences on acceptance of new ideas. Account Res 2008;15:30–62.
69. Schmaling KB, Blume AW. Ethics instruction increases graduate students' responsible conduct of research knowledge but not moral reasoning. Account Res 2009;16:268–83.
70. Plemmons DK, Brody S, Kalichman MW. Student perceptions of the effectiveness of education in the responsible conduct of research. Sci Eng Ethics 2006;12: 571–82.
71. Anderson MS, Horn AS, Risbey KR, et al. What do mentoring and training in the responsible conduct of research have to do with scientists' misbehavior? Finding from a national survey of NIH-funded scientists. Acad Med 2007;82:853–60.
72. Kalichman MW, Friedman PJ. A pilot study of biomedical trainees' perceptions concerning research ethics. Acad Med 1992;67:769–75.
73. Eastwood S, Derish P, Leash E, et al. Ethical issues in biomedical research: perceptions and practices of postdoctoral research fellows responding to a survey. Sci Eng Ethics 1996;2:89–114.
74. Price JH, Dake JA, Islam R. Selected ethical issues in research and publication: perceptions of health education faculty. Health Educ Behav 2011;28(1):51–64.
75. De Vries R, Anderson MS, Martinson BC. Normal misbehavior: scientists talk about the ethics of research. J Empir Res Hum Res Ethics 2006;1(1):43–50.
76. Martinson BC, Anderson MS, de Vries R. Scientists behaving badly. Nature 2005; 435:237–8.
77. Swazey J, Anderson MS, Lewis KS. Ethical problems in academic research. Am Sci 1993;81(6):542–53.
78. Titus SL. Evaluating U.S. medical schools' efforts to educate faculty researchers on research integrity and research misconduct policies and procedures. Account Res 2014;21:9–25.
79. Self DJ, Wolinsky FD, Baldwin DC Jr. The effect of teaching medical ethics on medical students' moral reasoning. Acad Med 1989;64:755–9.
80. Fleetwood J, Vaught W, Feldman D, et al. MedEthEx Online: a computer-based learning program in medical ethics and communication skills. Teach Learn Med 2000;12(2):96–104.

Interprofessional Musculoskeletal Education

A Review of National Initiatives from the Department of Veterans Affairs

Michael J. Battistone, MD[a],*, Andrea M. Barker, MPAS, PA-C[b],
Steven J. Durning, MD, PhD[c]

KEYWORDS

- Health professions education • Education • Continuing professional development
- Interprofessional education • Musculoskeletal education • Physical examination
- Clinical skills assessment • Procedural skills training

KEY POINTS

- The Department of Veterans Affairs (VA) created a portfolio of programs strengthening skills of primary care providers and health professions education (HPE) students and trainees in caring for veterans with musculoskeletal problems.
- Participants acquire an efficient and systematic approach to the physical examination of the shoulder and knee, which is easily incorporated into their daily practice.
- Program impact includes increased access to care and clinic services as well as reduction in unnecessary high-cost imaging.

Continued

Disclosure Statement: Disclosures: None to report.
Source of Funding: This work was supported by the United States Department of Veterans Affairs. This project was reviewed by the Institutional Review Board (IRB) of the University of Utah and Salt Lake City VA and was determined to be exempt from further IRB review because the work did not meet the definition of research with human subjects and was considered a quality improvement study.
Disclaimer: The views expressed in this article are those of the authors and do not necessarily reflect the official policy or position of the Uniformed Services University of the Health Sciences, the Department of Defense, or the Department of Veterans Affairs.

[a] Division of Rheumatology, Department of Medicine, Center of Excellence in Musculoskeletal Care and Education, George E. Wahlen Veterans Affairs Salt City Health Care System, University of Utah Health Sciences Center, Salt Lake City VA Medical Center, 11/E, 500 Foothill Drive, Salt Lake City, UT 84148, USA; [b] Department of Family and Preventive Medicine, Center of Excellence in Musculoskeletal Care and Education, George E. Wahlen Veterans Affairs Salt City Health Care System, University of Utah Health Sciences Center, Salt Lake City VA Medical Center, 11/E, 500 Foothill Drive, Salt Lake City, UT 84148, USA; [c] Graduate Programs in Health Professions Education, Uniformed Services University of the Health Sciences, 4301 Jones Bridge Road, Bethesda, MD 20814-4712, USA
* Corresponding author.
E-mail addresses: michael.battistone@va.gov; michael.battistone@hsc.utah.edu

Rheum Dis Clin N Am 46 (2020) 135–153
https://doi.org/10.1016/j.rdc.2019.09.004
0889-857X/20/Published by Elsevier Inc.

Continued

- The next steps are to expand these programs within the VA and other health care systems, and to enrich their impact, which will require the engagement of leaders and scholars in HPE.

INTRODUCTION

To address a gap in musculoskeletal (MSK) education, several recent initiatives have been launched, notably a series of national projects from the Department of Veterans Affairs (VA). The purpose of this review is to discuss the development of these VA MSK educational programs, their current state of operation, and the opportunities for additional MSK centers to become involved and to offer some suggestions for extending this work into other health care systems. In order to create a coherent understanding of why and how these VA programs were created, the authors begin by framing the background of the broader historical context in which they were developed. Second, the authors present summary descriptions of each program in the VA portfolio (**Table 1**), followed by a discussion of the goals, methods, and outcomes for each. These summaries will be of particular interest for readers engaged in health professions education (HPE) who are considering creating an initiative that will serve the range of HPE programs at their home institution. Third, the authors conclude by considering how this early work can be enhanced through additional scholarship undertaken in emerging VA–Department of Defense collaborations as well as the implications for the future of MSK education across the continuum of HPE and beyond the VA health care system.

Table 1 Portfolio of Veterans Affairs health professions musculoskeletal education programs			
Program	Learner Group	Length	Program Features
SLC Mini-Residency	PCP	1 wk Includes clinic	Evaluation and management of MSK issues common to primary care, including related procedural skills
National Mini-Residency	PCP	3 d ± Delayed clinic	Adapted content from SLC MR, deferred clinical experience to accommodate larger learner group Required partnership between SLC and training sites
COE MSK Education Week	HPE students and trainees	1 wk Includes clinic	Interprofessional and multidisciplinary group Core component of IM PGY1 ambulatory rotation
SimLEARN MSK Clinician	PCP	2 d No clinic	Shoulder and knee pain evaluation and management with simulation of relevant procedures
SimLEARN Master Educator	HPE clinical educators	2.5 d No clinic	Implementation of MSK program at home institution Creation of national consortium of MSK educators

Abbreviations: MR, mini-residency; SLC, Salt Lake City.

BACKGROUND

The development of the approaches to MSK education described in this article was driven by 3 influential factors:

1. An increased prioritization of MSK problems resulting from national reports and international initiatives,
2. A recognition that effective education for providers representing all health professions, not only physicians, was of critical importance in addressing these concerns,
3. The effectiveness of the VA in developing and sustaining innovative approaches to patient care and educational programs across the range of health professionals and the continuum of HPE.

International Efforts and National Reports

The Global Bone and Joint Decade (GBJD), one of the first international collaborative efforts to address a health concern in the twenty-first century, was launched by the World Health Organization in January 2000, in recognition of the significant impact of MSK disease worldwide.[1] This initiative, now known as the Global Alliance for Musculoskeletal Health, was influential in presenting a unified call to all nations to develop policies and practices addressing this problem within their particular health care systems.[2] Despite these efforts, MSK complaints continue to be the most frequent reason that patients seek medical attention, and recent data have estimated that the prevalence of MSK conditions has increased to more than 50%.[3–5]

In part because of the relative scarcity of rheumatologists, patients often seek care for MSK problems from their primary care providers (PCPs),[6] a cause for some concern because MSK training has been described as inadequate for these providers across the continuum of HPE in the United States and throughout the world.[6–14] The full effects of this situation are unknown; however, overutilization of high-cost imaging (ie, MRI) by PCPs is being recognized as a significant contributor to unnecessary health care spending.[15–17] The theme of this concern was so urgent that it became the subject of a 2012 report from the Institute of Medicine, *Best Care at Lower Cost: The Path to Continuously Learning Healthcare in America.*[18]

Importance of Musculoskeletal Education for All Health Professions Education Programs

In October 2011, the US Bone and Joint Initiative (USBJI, formed in 2002 as the US action group collaborating with the GBJD) held the first *Summit on the Value in Musculoskeletal Care.* The summary statement provided 15 recommendations, including a strong endorsement of the value of training across the spectrum of HPE:

"*Training programs for all health care providers should improve the knowledge, skills, and attitudes of all professionals in the diagnosis and management of musculoskeletal conditions. At present, many graduates report a deficit of knowledge of musculoskeletal conditions and competence in patient evaluation and treatment, including performance of the musculoskeletal physical examination.*"[19]

Effectiveness of Veterans Affairs

The success of the VA in developing effective responses can be attributed to 2 separate initiatives. First, in 2011, the VA issued a national call for proposals to expand veterans' access to health care services by providing new continuing professional development (CPD) programs for PCPs. These programs, described as "mini-residencies," were designed to strengthen PCPs' knowledge and skills in diagnosing and managing common primary care musculoskeletal (PC MSK) complaints. One of the overarching goals of the mini-residencies was to facilitate more appropriate use of specialty care resources. Second, in addition to these CPD programs, the VA used a competitive grant mechanism to create a limited number of "centers of excellence" to enhance clinical educational opportunities for HPE students and trainees rotating at VA medical centers affiliated with academic institutions. Through these 2 initiatives, the VA supported the efficient creation of effective MSK educational programs that can be delivered across the range of HPE learners, up to and including practicing providers. In addition, the relatively closed VA health care system provides unique opportunities to examine long-term consequences of these educational programs on provider behavior, and ultimately, on the veterans' experience and the quality of care. Both of these outcomes have important implications for MSK care and for considering new models of clinical education and training in other health care systems in the United States.

Cost-Effectiveness Projection

The first step in the development of the programs described in later discussion was an analysis of projected cost-effectiveness of an educational intervention designed to train PCPs to perform knee injections in their local clinics.[20] The authors anticipated that this would be most relevant for VA providers in rural settings, where patients would otherwise have to travel long distances to receive care. Although distance from the PCP to the referral center was a factor, the number of patients was the primary driver of cost-effectiveness, even if the clinic was within 50 miles of the center. The analysis projected that an educational program would be cost-effective if at least 20 patients with knee pain, in whom an injection would be appropriate to consider, were seen each year by the trained provider at their site. These findings informed the development and assessment of the programs now described.

DESCRIPTIONS OF PROGRAMS
Salt Lake City Musculoskeletal Mini-Residency

Goals
The primary purpose of this program was to strengthen the ability of PCPs to effectively evaluate and manage shoulder and knee pain, including providing joint injections when indicated, in the primary care setting.[21] Because this was the first program developed, it also served as the template that informed the construction of subsequent MSK educational initiatives described in later discussion.

Methods
The first course began April 23, 2012 and was held periodically on the campus of the George E. Wahlen Salt Lake City VA, through September 2013. Opportunity to participate was communicated directly to PCPs through VA e-mail, and to regional administrators and clinical leaders on conference calls throughout VA. Potential participants completed a brief application; key factors considered in determining acceptance to the training program included the burden of MSK disease in applicants' clinic population, limited availability of other MSK specialty providers able to perform procedures, and the participants' anticipation of how the training would impact their clinical practice. Participants' costs for travel and living expenses (average estimated cost per participant was $2000) were supported by VA Specialty Care Services/Specialty Care Transformation, Office of Patient Care Services (SCS/SCT, OPCS). This experience was accredited by the VA Employee Education System for 40 hours of category 1 CPD credit.

General program description In its initial form, the Salt Lake City MSK "mini-residency" was a 2-week event, although in order to accommodate the large number of PCPs interested in the training, the number of course offerings were increased by condensing the program to 1 week. The schedule for this final iteration of the MSK mini-residency is provided in **Fig. 1**. The overall approach was informed by Kolb's theory of experiential learning cycles, in which *abstract conceptualization* (didactics) is followed by *active experimentation* (peer-assisted learning of physical examination components), then by *concrete experiences* (supervised clinical experiences with actual patients), and concluding with *reflective observation* (course debriefing and structured self- and objective assessments with feedback).[22] In constructing the course, the authors followed the 6-step model of curriculum development outlined by Kern and colleagues[23] and Thomas and colleagues.[24]

The fourth step of the Kern and Thomas model involves the consideration of educational strategies. In this, the authors recognize the specific contributions of O'Dunn-Orto, Berman, and Monrad, whose work emphasized the value of small-group, interactive sessions, peer-learning techniques, simulation, direct supervision, task decomposition, and varied emphasis techniques in optimizing transfer of MSK clinical skills.[11,12,25]

Shoulder and knee physical examination Primary objectives of the program included strengthening participants' confidence and competence in the physical examination of the shoulder and knee. These objectives were congruent with USBJI recommendations and were also identified by participants as one of the most valued elements of the training. In building this portion of the curriculum, a systematic process was used to define elements of a specialty-level physical examination that were also feasible for PCPs to use in their clinics, and to develop an efficient and systematic method of teaching and assessing these. Rather than using a "diagnosis-driven" approach, the conceptual framework for the examination maneuvers was grounded in the anatomy of the shoulder and knee. Two rheumatologists, 2 orthopedic surgeons, and a physician assistant with an orthopedic background proposed sets of specific observable examination maneuvers as well as criteria that would guide faculty raters in assessing the quality with which each maneuver was performed. These sets were further informed through literature review, finalized by consensus, and organized into sequential checklists to operationalize the examination sequences. These checklists (**Figs. 2** and **3**) are provided in the course syllabus, which is supplemented by online video content demonstrating the performance of the complete examinations.[26,27] Details regarding the construction of these materials, including an expanded formal consensus project and other evidence of validity, have been presented elsewhere.[28,29]

Osteoporosis Basic concepts, including risk factors, current screening recommendations, definitions, and diagnosis of osteopenia and osteoporosis, as well as appropriate treatment options were discussed in small group sessions facilitated by an endocrinologist.

Arthrocentesis/joint injections MSK procedures (knee aspiration and injection, and subacromial space injection) were taught using the "No Touch" technique described by Wittich and colleagues.[30] All aspects, indications, contraindications, informed consent, patient positioning, identification, and disinfection of the injection site, and the procedural technique itself, were presented by an orthopedist; this was followed by supervised practice sessions using simulation task trainers.

	Day 1	Day 2	Day 3	Day 4	Day 5
	Pre-course Assessment				
	Shoulder Physical Examination	Knee Physical Examination	Rheum Topics in Primary Care Part I	Orthopedic Injection Clinic	Musculoskeletal Multidisciplinary Center of Excellence Clinic
			Knee Skills Assessment (OSCE)		
	Shoulder Physical Examination	Knee Physical Examination	Rheum Topics in Primary Care Part II		
	Shoulder Pathology	Knee Pathology			
	Lunch	Lunch	Lunch	Lunch	Lunch
	Shoulder Cases	Arthrocentesis – Shoulder and Knee	Osteoporosis: Additional Risk Factors	Primary Care MSK Clinic	Rheumatoid Arthritis Clinic
		Knee Cases & Arthrocentesis Practice			
	Osteoporosis: Definitions, Diagnosis, and Risk Factors -Didactic and Case Presentation-	Osteoporosis: Treatment	Back Pain in Primary Care		Post-course Assessment
		Shoulder Skills Assessment (OSCE)			

Didactic   Small Group Practice   Clinic Experiences   Assessments

Fig. 1. Salt Lake City 5-day MSK Mini-Residency program schedule.

Shoulder Physical Examination

	Examination Item	Performed	Adequate Technique
1	*Observation*		
	Exposure	0 1 2	Observe as they disrobe for discomfort
	General posterior observation	0 1 2	Symmetry, scars, lesions, atrophy
	Scapular winging/dyskinesia	0 1 2	Patient raises arms bilaterally; wall press
2	*Palpation*		
	Sternoclavicular joints	0 1 2	
	Acromioclavicular joints	0 1 2	
	Biceps tendons	0 1 2	
	Subacromial space	0 1 2	Lateral and posterolateral
3	*Range of Motion (ROM)*		
4	*Motor Function of Rotator Cuff*		
	Bilateral		

Supraspinatus	ROM: Active abduction in scapular plane
	  Painful arc (>90°)
	  Drop arm test
		0 1 2	Scapular plane, neutral rotation
			Allow for full active adduction

Supraspinatus	Motor: Empty Can Test	0 1 2	Scapular plane, full pronation Resisted abduction lower than 90°
Infraspinatus	ROM: Active external rotation	0 1 2	Elbows at side
Infraspinatus	Motor: Active external rotation against resistance	0 1 2	Elbows at side Start with hands near midline
	Unilateral		
Subscapularis	Motor: Belly Press Test	0 1 2	Hand on abdomen, elbow anterior to midline Examiner pulls at forearm Watch for elbow to drop
Subscapularis	ROM: Active internal rotation along spine	0 1 2	Observe patient from behind
Subscapularis	Motor: Lift Off Test	0 1 2	Hand at lumbar spine Actively lifts arm off back, resistance at wrist
Teres Minor	ROM: Active external rotation with 90° shoulder abduction and 90° elbow flexion	*0 1 2*	90° shoulder abduction & 90° elbow flexion Active external rotation
Teres Minor	Motor: Hornblower's Test	0 1 2	External rotation as above against resistance
	Note: Check passive ROM if active is limited. This will help identify a mechanical block versus weakness or pain		
5	*Provocative Testing*		
	Impingement Testing		
	Hawkin's Test	0 1 2	Shoulder 90° abduction in scapular plane 90° elbow flexion, internal rotation + horizontal adduction
	Neer's Test	0 1 2	Elbow extended, arm in full pronation Maximal passive forward elevation of shoulder with scapular stabilization
	Biceps Testing		
	Speed's Test	0 1 2	Hand in supination 60° forward elevation, 20-30° elbow flexion Apply downward pressure to forearm
	Yergason's Test	0 1 2	Elbow at side, 90° flexion; palm in supination Resisted supination
	Acromioclavicular Joint Testing		
	Cross-arm Test	0 1 2	Active horizontal adduction
	Scoring: 0 = Item not performed. 1 = Item performed but technique not adequate. 2 = Item performed correctly.		

Fig. 2. Shoulder physical examination checklist.

Inflammatory arthropathies This portion of the curriculum provided time for a review of inflammatory joint diseases, including gout, rheumatoid arthritis (RA), and spondyloarthropathies. These topics were discussed in small groups facilitated by a rheumatologist; particular emphasis was given to conversations regarding high-value use of laboratory testing in primary care settings.

Knee Physical Examination

	Examination Item	Performed	Adequate Technique
1	*Observation*		
	Standing	0 1 2	Gait, alignment, popliteal fossa
	Supine position, knee adequately exposed	0 1 2	Alignment, atrophy, erythema, scar
	Effusion	0 1 2	Full extension. Check medial & lateral gutters
2	*Range of Motion*		
	Extension and Flexion (0-140°)	0 1 2	
	Hip IR (30°) and ER (60°)	0 1 2	Keep femur perpendicular to floor
3	*Palpation*		
	Flex to 90° with heel resting on table	0 1 2	Take time between each landmark Use sufficient pressure
	Quadriceps tendon	0 1 2	
	Patellar tendon	0 1 2	
	Tibial tubercle	0 1 2	
	Lateral joint line	0 1 2	
	Lateral femoral epicondyle (proximal LCL)	0 1 2	
	Fibular head (distal LCL)	0 1 2	
	Medial joint line	0 1 2	
	Medial femoral epicondyle (proximal MCL)	0 1 2	
	Medial tibial plateau (distal MCL)	0 1 2	
	Pes anserine bursa	0 1 2	
4	*Stability Testing*		
	Posterior Cruciate Ligament Posterior Drawer	0 1 2	Knee flexed to 90 degrees Examiner stabilizes foot Thumbs on anterior tibia, translate posterior
	Anterior Cruciate Ligament Anterior drawer	0 1 2	Knee flexed to 90 degrees Examiner stabilizes foot Thumbs on anterior tibia, translate anterior
	Anterior Cruciate Ligament Lachman Test	0 1 2	Knee flexed to 30 degrees Hands near joint line Anterior tibial translation
	Medial Collateral Ligament Valgus stress	0 1 2	30 degrees flexion
	Lateral Collateral Ligament Varus stress	0 1 2	30 degrees flexion
5	*Provocative Testing*		
	Meniscus Testing		
	Medial Meniscus McMurray Test	0 1 2	Fingers on medial joint line Full knee flexion Thumb/heel point medial = tibia external rotation Varus stress and slow knee extension
	Lateral Meniscus McMurray Test	0 1 2	Fingers on lateral joint line Full knee flexion Thumb/heel point lateral = tibial internal rotation Valgus stress and slow knee extension
	Patellofemoral Assessment		
	Palpation of medial and lateral patellar facets	0 1 2	Knee in extension
	Patellar Compression Test	0 1 2	Active quadriceps contraction Repeated with posterior patellar compression
	IT Band Assessment		
	Noble Compression Test	0 1 2	Palpate lateral femoral epicondyle Passive knee ROM with pain around 30°
Scoring: 0 = Item not performed. 1 = Item performed but technique not adequate. 2 = Item performed correctly.			

Fig. 3. Knee physical examination checklist.

Clinical experiences The didactic and peer-practice sessions in the first part of the week facilitated learners' tasks of abstract conceptualization and active experimentation; this prepared them for the concrete experiences and reflective observation with faculty in 4 settings: an orthopedic injection clinic, a PC MSK clinic, a dedicated RA clinic, and a multidisciplinary MSK clinic where complex cases were evaluated and managed by all faculty (more detail regarding these clinics is presented in later discussion). In preparation for their active engagement in the clinic environment, learners completed the local credentialing process required for these experiences. Participants elicited history, conducted examinations, interpreted findings, discussed management options, and, when appropriate, performed procedures, all under direct supervision of faculty.

Outcomes

Each week-long course included up to 4 PCPs; from April 2012 through September 2013, a total of 38 providers participated, representing 32 clinics from 15 states (**Table 2**).

An early observation of the initial participants in the MSK mini-residency demonstrated a progressive increase in the number of joint injections performed by program alumni at their local clinics in the months following their training.[21] Joint injection rates has been confirmed after 2 years of follow-up using the entire cohort of participants; a preliminary analysis of these data has been presented, and the manuscript is in preparation.[31] The authors also have reported other examples of change in practice behavior, notably a reduction in unnecessary MRIs ordered by course participants.[32]

A third meaningful outcome was the substantial interest in this type of training that was demonstrated by PCPs, indicated by the rising number of applications received relative to the number of opportunities available. Despite doubling the number of course offerings, and the number of participants included in each course, the authors simply were not able to satisfy the demand for this experience. Learner interest in this experience was the primary factor in developing a new educational model, the National MSK Mini-Residency, which is discussed later.[33]

National Musculoskeletal Mini-Residency

Goals

This program was supported by the VA central office (OSCS), with the goal of disseminating the successful local Salt Lake City MSK Mini-Residency as broadly as possible, while preserving consistency in teaching and evaluation of learners' competence.[33] The primary objectives were to

Table 2
Health professionals trained in Veterans Affairs musculoskeletal education programs from 2012 to 2019

		Profession				
	Physician	Physician Assistant	Nurse Practitioner	Nurse	Other	Total
CPD programs						
SLC MR	26	1	11			38
National MR	135	21	61	10		227
National SLC MR	25	6	20	1	1	53
SimLEARN MSK C	46	10	19	1	1	77
SimLEARN MSK ME	29	1	6			36
Total	*261*	*39*	*117*	*12*	*2*	*431*
Student & Trainee Program						
Student	28	75	41		1	145
Resident	337				14	351
Fellow	15					15
Total	*380*	*75*	*41*	*0*	*15*	*511*
Grand Total	*641*	*114*	*158*	*12*	*17*	*942*

1. Increase the capacity of the Salt Lake City MSK Mini-Residency so that more PCPs could be trained in less time,
2. Strengthen participants' confidence in the physical examination of the shoulder and knee,
3. Document their competence through an objective structured clinical examination (OSCE).

High fidelity of this experience was ensured through the participation of 2 course faculty staffing each OSCE station: one as simulated patient and the other as rater.[29] The OSCE was meant to serve as a proxy for sufficient preparation for participation in subsequent clinical experiences that could be provided at a later date. This experience was accredited by the VA Employee Education System for 24 hours of category 1 CPD credit.

Methods
Creation of educational partnerships Sites were selected on the basis of their response to a request for proposals from OSCS, in which they identified 2 local HPE leaders: 1 rheumatologist and 1 generalist, to work with Salt Lake City faculty in preparing and presenting a mini-residency program at their local institution. Leaders from approved sites traveled to Salt Lake City for a brief "train-the-trainer" program to introduce the curriculum and methods of teaching as well as learner assessment.

General program description The schedule of the National MSK Mini-Residency consisted of only the first 3 days of the 5-day Salt Lake City program (see **Fig. 1**). To accommodate the larger numbers of participants at each national program, as well as site-specific variations in weekly clinic schedules, local faculty worked with learners after the 3-day mini-residency to arrange supervised clinical experiences in which this training could be applied.

Outcomes
Over the 2 years of the National MSK Mini-Residency (2012–2014), programs were presented at 13 sites. Two hundred twenty-seven learners participated in the training, 212 of whom (93%) also completed the OSCEs (see **Table 2**). The mean OSCE score was 90% for the shoulder and 86% for knee, which the authors interpret as an indicator of effective skill acquisition for most of our learners.[33] This 3-day National MSK-Mini-Residency course continues to be offered twice yearly at the Salt Lake City VA, with the possibility of extending the experience to include the supervised clinic experiences, which were part of the original week-long program.

Center of Excellence in Musculoskeletal Care and Education

Goals
Although the mini-residencies targeted the educational needs of *practicing providers*, the goal of the MSK Center of Excellence (COE) was to strengthen knowledge and skills of *HPE students and trainees*, with an emphasis on learning and working in an interdisciplinary and interprofessional health care system.[34] To this end, 2 new MSK clinics and an intensive week-long experience, the "MSK Education Week," were created.

Methods
The structure of this experience, implemented in 2012, shares the same theoretic underpinning as the Salt Lake City MSK Mini-Residency, as well as a similar 5-day schedule. Documentation of participants' competence using the 2-station OSCE described above occurs midweek, following the didactic and physical examination

practice sessions, before the clinical experiences in the latter half of the curriculum. An additional OSCE station simulating preparation for and performance of an intraarticular knee injection was developed to further prepare learners to participate with faculty in performing procedures in the clinics.[35]

One unique feature of the MSK Education Week is its integration with the core curricula of several HPE programs at the University of Utah, the academic affiliate of the Salt Lake City VA. This integration is reflected in the frequency with which this program is offered, and the advance planning which is required, 1 week each month is reserved for the MSK Education Week, and specific dates are projected 2 years in advance.

Participants The learner group, HPE students and trainees, is another unique feature distinguishing this program from the others in the VA portfolio. Participants are selected from those who have been scheduled by their specific training program for VA clinic rotations during the time in which an Education Week is being conducted. The Week has become a core program requirement for all postgraduate year (PGY) 1 categorical internal medicine (IM) residents, "preliminary" neurology and physical medicine and rehabilitation (PM&R) residents, and PGY 3 residents in family and preventive medicine. Fourth-year medical students, as well as students from the physician assistant and nurse practitioner programs, and residents and fellows from other disciplines can participate on a space-available basis and receive academic credit for an elective experience. The total number of learners per week ranges between 8 and 10, limited by the capacity to provide a sufficient number of clinical experiences.

Clinical experiences Two new-model MSK clinics were developed as part of the COE–the PC MSK Clinic and the multidisciplinary MSK COE clinic, offering hands-on application of the skills learned during the first half of the MSK Education Week.

The PC MSK Clinic is a high-volume, procedurally heavy clinic embedded within primary care and staffed by 2 rheumatologists and a physician assistant with orthopedic experience. Using a consult request within the VA electronic medical record, the Computerized Patient Record System, patients are referred for focused evaluation and management of common MSK conditions, typically those involving the shoulder (primarily partial and full-thickness rotator cuff tears, osteoarthritis, and adhesive capsulitis), and the knee (mainly osteoarthritis and patellofemoral pain syndrome). After a comprehensive history and physical examination are performed, learners will discuss the case with clinic faculty and perform related joint and soft tissue injections under direct supervision, when indicated.

The multidisciplinary MSK COE clinic focuses on patients with more complex conditions, as well as those who have not had satisfying results through traditional specialty care systems using a team of providers from rheumatology, endocrinology, orthopedics, PM&R, and primary care. Learners independently evaluate a patient and then present the case to the team, followed by a group discussion. At the conclusion of the visit, both the patient and the learner will have interacted with multiple disciplines to create an appropriate care plan.

Outcomes

The MSK Education Week is conducted each month, engaging a diverse group of interprofessional students and trainees from the range of HPE programs (**Fig. 4**). Since the inaugural event in April 2012, more than 500 learners have participated; the substantial increase in numbers began in the second year of the program (**Table 3**), when the authors' training experience was integrated as an element of the IM PGY 1 core curriculum, a required VA ambulatory care rotation.

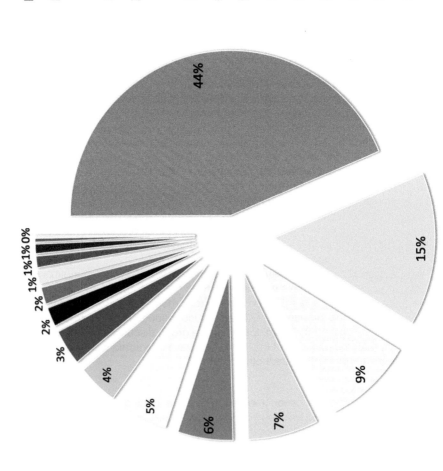

Fig. 4. Interprofessional and interdisciplinary cohort of 511 learners from the COE Musculoskeletal Education Week, 2012 to 2019.

Table 3
Center of Excellence musculoskeletal education week programs and participants from 2012 to 2019

Academic Year	Number of Program Offerings	Number of Participants	Average Number of Participants per Program
2012–2013	5	23	5
2013–2014	11	71	6
2014–2015	11	82	7
2015–2016	12	82	7
2016–2017	11	80	7
2017–2018	12	87	7
2018–2019	11	86	8
Total	73	511	

Increased clinical productivity is another important outcome of this program. **Fig. 5** shows the numbers of patient encounters in the PC MSK and MSK COE clinics from the time they were established. Each encounter represents a clinical training opportunity for a student or trainee, and approximately 50% of the encounters in the PC MSK clinic involved a procedure that the learner performed under supervision.

The clinics offer additional learning opportunities for rheumatology fellows, as these weekly experiences have become part of their VA rotation schedule. The relatively high number of joint aspirations and injections performed in the PC MSK clinic, as well as the opportunity to be supervised by orthopedic and PM&R attendings in the MSK COE clinic, facilitates their own procedural skill acquisition. Moreover, participation by junior trainees during the MSK Weeks provides unique teaching opportunities for fellows in the ambulatory setting.

Finally, the establishment of the MSK Week and associated clinics has created many opportunities for HPE scholarship. These opportunities have included projects exploring cognitive load during procedural training, clinical reasoning in the context of decisions regarding the use of high-cost imaging, and an interinstitutional

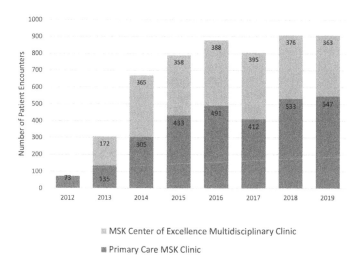

■ MSK Center of Excellence Multidisciplinary Clinic

■ Primary Care MSK Clinic

Fig. 5. Increase in clinical productivity for the COE MSK clinics, 2012 to 2019.

collaborative project with Siaton and colleagues[36,37] addressing the feasibility of implementing a script concordance test for gout that had been previously created and studied at another institution and context.

Simulation Learning, Education, and Research Network National Simulation Center Musculoskeletal Training Programs

Goals

The recently constructed Veterans Health Affairs (VHA) Simulation Learning, Education, and Research Network (SimLEARN) National Simulation Center in Orlando, Florida was created with the goal of development and delivery of simulation-based training curricula to facilitate VA workforce CPD.[38] Following the success of the national 3-day MSK mini-residency experience, leaders from SimLEARN worked with mini-residency faculty to create 2 recurring MSK training programs: the MSK Clinician (MSK C) and the MSK Master Educator (MSK ME) (Barker AM, LaRochelle JL, Artino AR, et al. The veterans health Affairs simulation learning, education and research network [SimLEARN] national musculoskeletal training programs: new resources and career development opportunities for primary care providers and leaders in health professions education. Submitted for publication).

The goals of the MSK C are the same as for those of the National MSK Mini-Residency: to strengthen PCPs' confidence in their ability to perform high-level physical examinations of the shoulder and knee and to document learners' competence in the OSCE. This training also provides preparation to participate in MSK procedure clinics, if the goal of the individual PCP is to become credentialed to perform joint aspirations or injections.

The MSK ME is a faculty development course, developed for those with preexisting MSK content knowledge and experience who are interested in implementing an MSK educational program at their home institution, and who would value the introduction to a national curriculum and participation in a community of practice and teaching with other MSK MEs. The MSK C and MSK ME courses are accredited by the VA Employee Education System for 16 and 20 hours of category 1 CPD credit, respectively.

Methods

The 2-day MSK C schedule mirrors the national program for the shoulder and knee content: didactic presentation, small group peer-learning, simulation case-based learning, and evaluations of competence through an OSCE. Participants are observed performing simulated joint injections of the subacromial space and intraarticular knee on task-trainers, with concomitant faculty guidance and feedback. These experiences prepare participants for subsequent injections on actual patients at their home institution, supervised by a provider who is currently credentialed to perform the same procedure.

The MSK ME program schedule is shown in **Fig. 6**. Clinical educators are presented with the MSK C curriculum and the approach the authors have described in teaching this content to PCPs and HPE students and trainees. On the second day of the program, MSK ME learners participate in the OSCE, both to assess their command of the elements in the examination checklists and to familiarize them with the OSCE process from the learner's perspective. Throughout the course, instructors encourage participant feedback on the curriculum and facilitate discussions of what an effective MSK educational program would look like at their own institutions, and how it might be best launched. On the final day, course participants take part in a 3-station objective structured teaching experience (OSTE), in which they rotate through assigned roles of

Day 1	Day 2	Day 3
Pre-course Assessment	Knee Physical Examination	Observed Structured Teaching Experience (OSTE)
Shoulder Physical Examination		
	Knee Physical Examination	
Shoulder Physical Examination	Knee Pathology	OSTE Debriefing
Shoulder Pathology	Knee Injections	Implementation & Scholarship Group Discussion
	Knee Injections	
Lunch	Lunch	Post-course Assessment
Shoulder Cases	Knee Cases	
Arthrocentesis Introduction & Shoulder Injections	Implementation & Local Planning	
Shoulder Injections		
Review Current Literature in MSK Education	Knee and Shoulder Skills Assessment (OSCE)	

Fig. 6. Schedule for the SimLEARN Master Educator program.

learner, rater, and simulated patient. Immediately following each rotation, course faculty conducts debriefing sessions. This method of faculty development, especially when combined with focused group debriefing, has been described as being both effective and acceptable.[39–43]

Outcomes

As the SimLEARN courses are the most recent additions to the VA portfolio, outcome data are limited. To date, 10 MSK C and 6 MSK ME courses have been conducted with up to 75 clinicians having participated (see **Table 2**). A greater demand for MSK C courses is anticipated, because of the higher numbers of clinicians in the VHA system, compared with HPE educators. To address the need for qualified faculty to teach these MSK C courses, participants completing the MSK ME pathway may be invited to become instructors for MSK C programs. Opportunities such as these facilitate further development of an interprofessional, and interinstitutional, community of MSK educators: a valuable resource for the ongoing maintenance and refinement of these existing courses as well as the creation of new educational initiatives and programs of study for HPE.

FUTURE DIRECTIONS

Two questions, broadly addressing the quantity and quality of impact, help to frame the discussion of potential next steps for this work. First, how can the context for similarly successful programs for MSK education be *expanded*? This question has implications not only for additional VA centers but also for other government health care structures, such as the Public Health Service and Military Health System, which, like the VA, also seek to optimize access to appropriate care and provide career development opportunities that are fit for purpose. Furthermore, although the work the authors have described has occurred within the unique environment of the VA, the lessons learned in developing and adapting the curriculum to produce several variations on a theme are applicable to other nonprofit or private health care systems, particularly those that seek to strengthen cost-conscious, high-value care for common MSK problems.

The second question refers to the quality, the character, of these programs: how can the impact of this work be *enriched*? This question is more complex. Although it is important to seek evidence demonstrating *that* interventions worked, a more fundamental task is to search for explanations as to *why* they did or did not work. Careful, rigorous scholarship will be essential in these efforts. In addition to examining effects of training on quality improvement indicators, HPE research seeks to strengthen all HPE by increasing our understanding of how we learn.[44–46]

SUMMARY

The authors have reviewed several recent initiatives in MSK education that have been developed for learners across disciplines and along the continuum of HPE and training pathways. In addition, there are opportunities for educational leaders in rheumatology, as well as in primary care, to contribute to the continued refinement of the national curriculum and to collaborate in the scholarship that will be necessary in constructing educational programs fit for the purpose of ensuring a well-trained, competent workforce of health care providers.

REFERENCES

1. Woolf AD. The bone and joint decade. Strategies to reduce the burden of disease: the Bone and Joint Monitor Project. J Rheumatol Suppl 2003;67:6–9.
2. Woolf AD, Gabriel S. Overcoming challenges in order to improve the management of rheumatic and musculoskeletal diseases across the globe. Clin Rheumatol 2015;34(5):815–7.
3. Cherry DK, Hing E, Woodwell DA, Rechtsteiner EA. National Ambulatory Medical Care Survey: 2006 survey. Natl Health Stat Report 2008;6(3):1–39.
4. Yelin E, Weinstein S, King T. The burden of musculoskeletal diseases in the United States. Semin Arthritis Rheum 2016;46(3):259–60.
5. Goulet JL, Kerns RD, Bair M, et al. The musculoskeletal diagnosis cohort: examining pain and pain care among veterans. Pain 2016;157(8):1696–703.
6. FitzGerald JD, Battistone M, Brown CR Jr, et al. Regional distribution of adult rheumatologists. Arthritis Rheum 2013;65(12):3017–25.
7. Glazier RH, Dalby DM, Badley EM, et al. Determinants of physician confidence in the primary care management of musculoskeletal disorders. J Rheumatol 1996; 23(2):351–6.

8. Houston TK, Connors RL, Cutler N, et al. A primary care musculoskeletal clinic for residents: success and sustainability. J Gen Intern Med 2004;19(5 Pt 2):524–9.
9. Day CS, Yeh AC. Evidence of educational inadequacies in region-specific musculoskeletal medicine. Clin Orthop Relat Res 2008;466(10):2542–7.
10. Haywood BL, Porter SL, Grana WA. Assessment of musculoskeletal knowledge in primary care residents. Am J Orthop (Belle Mead NJ) 2006;35(6):273–5.
11. Monrad SU, Zeller JL, Craig CL, et al. Musculoskeletal education in US medical schools: lessons from the past and suggestions for the future. Curr Rev Musculoskelet Med 2011;4(3):91–8.
12. O'Dunn-Orto A, Hartling L, Campbell S, et al. Teaching musculoskeletal clinical skills to medical trainees and physicians: a Best Evidence in Medical Education systematic review of strategies and their effectiveness: BEME Guide No. 18. Med Teach 2012;34(2):93–102.
13. Smith CC, Newman L, Davis RB, et al. A comprehensive new curriculum to teach and assess resident knowledge and diagnostic evaluation of musculoskeletal complaints. Med Teach 2005;27(6):553–8.
14. Wilcox T, Oyler J, Harada C, et al. Musculoskeletal exam and joint injection training for internal medicine residents. J Gen Intern Med 2006;21(5):521–3.
15. Petron DJ, Greis PE, Aoki SK, et al. Use of knee magnetic resonance imaging by primary care physicians in patients aged 40 years and older. Sports Health 2010;2(5):385–90.
16. Roberts TT, Singer N, Hushmendy S, et al. MRI for the evaluation of knee pain: comparison of ordering practices of primary care physicians and orthopaedic surgeons. J Bone Joint Surg Am 2015;97(9):709–14.
17. Wylie JD, Crim JR, Working ZM, et al. Physician provider type influences utilization and diagnostic utility of magnetic resonance imaging of the knee. J Bone Joint Surg Am 2015;97(1):56–62.
18. Smith MD, Institute of Medicine (U.S.), Committee on the Learning Health Care System in America. Best care at lower cost: the path to continuously learning health care in America. Washington, DC: National Academies Press; 2013.
19. Gnatz SM, Pisetsky DS, Andersson GB. The value in musculoskeletal care: summary and recommendations. Semin Arthritis Rheum 2012;41(5):741–4.
20. Nelson RE, Battistone MJ, Ashworth WD, et al. Cost effectiveness of training rural providers to perform joint injections. Arthritis Care Res (Hoboken) 2014;66(4):559–66.
21. Battistone MJ, Barker AM, Lawrence P, et al. Mini-residency in musculoskeletal care: an interprofessional, mixed-methods educational initiative for primary care providers. Arthritis Care Res (Hoboken) 2016;68(2):275–9.
22. Kolb DA. Experiential learning: experience as the source of learning and development. Englewood Cliffs (NJ): Prentice-Hall; 1984.
23. Kern DE, Thomas PA, Hughes MT. Curriculum development for medical education: a six-step approach. 2nd edition. Baltimore (MD): Johns Hopkins University Press; 2009.
24. Thomas PA, Kern DE, Hughes MT, et al. Curriculum development for medical education: a six-step approach. 3rd edition. Baltimore (MD): Johns Hopkins University Press; 2016.
25. Berman JR, Ben-Artzi A, Fisher MC, et al. A comparison of arthrocentesis teaching tools: cadavers, synthetic joint models, and the relative utility of different educational modalities in improving trainees' comfort with procedures. J Clin Rheumatol 2012;18(4):175–9.

26. Barker AM, Battistone MJ. Shoulder physical exam. 2015. Available at: https://www.youtube.com/watch?v=dzHFwkXBmvU. Accessed October 6, 2019.

27. Barker AM, Battistone MJ. Knee physical exam for primary care providers. 2015. Available at: https://www.youtube.com/watch?v=YhYrMisCrWA. Accessed October 6, 2019.

28. Barker AM, Brahaj A, Carvalho P, et al. Development of musculoskeletal physical examination checklists: a formal consensus project involving national educators. Arthritis Rheum 2017;69.

29. Battistone MJ, Barker AM, Beck JP, et al. Validity evidence for two objective structured clinical examination stations to evaluate core skills of the shoulder and knee assessment. BMC Med Educ 2017;17(1):13.

30. Wittich CM, Ficalora RD, Mason TG, et al. Musculoskeletal injection. Mayo Clin Proc 2009;84(9):831–6 [quiz: 837].

31. Battistone MJ, Barker AM, Lawrence P, et al. Two-year impact of a continuing professional education program to train primary care providers to perform arthrocentesis. Arthritis Rheum 2017;69(suppl 10).

32. Call MR, Barker AM, Lawrence P, et al. Impact of a musculoskeletal "mini-residency" continuing professional education program on knee MRI orders by primary care providers. Arthritis Rheum 2015;67(suppl 10).

33. Battistone MJ, Barker AM, Grotzke MP, et al. "Mini-residency" in musculoskeletal care: a national continuing professional development program for primary care providers. J Gen Intern Med 2016;31(11):1301–7.

34. Battistone MJ, Barker AM, Grotzke MP, et al. Effectiveness of an interprofessional and multidisciplinary musculoskeletal training program. J Grad Med Educ 2016; 8(3):398–404.

35. Braaten T, Barker AM, Beck JP, et al. Validity evidence for an objective structured clinical examination station to assess knee arthrocentesis skill. Arthritis Rheum 2017;69(suppl 10).

36. Siaton BC, Clayton E, Kueider AM, et al. Use of script concordance testing to evaluate the efficacy of a web-based module on gout: three years of experience. Arthritis Rheumatol 2016;68(suppl 10).

37. Siaton BC, Barker AM, Battistone MJ. A pilot study of the use of a validated gout script concordance test assessment in an interdisciplinary musculoskeletal education program. Arthritis Rheumatol 2017;69(suppl 10).

38. Available at: https://www.simlearn.va.gov/SIMLEARN/about_us.asp. Accessed October 6, 2019.

39. Macedo L, Sturpe DA, Haines ST, et al. An objective structured teaching exercise (OSTE) for preceptor development. Curr Pharm Teach Learn 2015;7:627–34.

40. McCutcheon LRM, Whitcomb K, Cox CD, et al. Interprofessional objective structured teaching exercise (iOSTE) to train preceptors. Curr Pharm Teach Learn 2017;9(4):605–15.

41. Steinert Y, Mann K, Centeno A, et al. A systematic review of faculty development initiatives designed to improve teaching effectiveness in medical education: BEME Guide No. 8. Med Teach 2006;28(6):497–526.

42. Sturpe D, Schaivone KA. Regarding use of objective structured teaching exercises (OSTE) for summative evaluations (authors' response). Am J Pharm Educ 2015;79(5):73.

43. Sturpe DA, Schaivone KA. A primer for objective structured teaching exercises. Am J Pharm Educ 2014;78(5):104.

44. Kanter SL. Toward better descriptions of innovations. Acad Med 2008;83(8): 703–4.
45. Haji F, Morin MP, Parker K. Rethinking programme evaluation in health professions education: beyond 'did it work?'. Med Educ 2013;47(4):342–51.
46. Cianciolo AT, Regehr G. Learning theory and educational intervention: producing meaningful evidence of impact through layered analysis. Acad Med 2019;94(6): 789–94.

Education and Professional Development in Rheumatology

Translating Quality Improvement and Education to Clinical Practice

Christina Downey, MD, RhMSUS[a],*, Deepa Ragesh Panikkath, MD[a],
Daniel H. Solomon, MD, MPH[b,c]

KEYWORDS

• Quality improvement • Fellowship training • Rheumatology • Academic milestones

KEY POINTS

- Rheumatology fellows are expected to learn how to improve the quality of the care they provide by the end of their fellowship and should be able to expand this to a systems-based approach.
- Faculty may not be equipped to provide quality improvement (QI) teaching to fellows.
- Learning by doing is a suitable and effective way to teach QI.
- There are resources available to assist both faculty and fellows in completing QI processes.
- Fellows offer unique perspectives on patient care and their input can improve the care delivery to patients at their respective organizations.

INTRODUCTION

In March 2010, the Affordable Care Act (ACA) was passed, bringing with it an increased focus on the cost and delivery of health care. Two of the 3 goals of the ACA directly pertain to quality improvement (QI): to control costs of health care, and

C. Downey and D. Unni: The authors have no potential conflicts to declare. D.H. Solomon: Support: NIH-P30-AR072577 (VERITY). Potential Conflicts: The author receives salary support from research contracts to his institution from AbbVie, Amgen, Corrona, Genentech, and Janssen.
[a] Division of Rheumatology, Loma Linda University Medical Center, 11234 Anderson Street, Loma Linda, CA 92354, USA; [b] Division of Rheumatology, Immunology and Allergy, Brigham and Women's Hospital, Harvard Medical School, 75 Francis Street, Boston, MA 02115, USA; [c] Division of Pharmacoepidemiology, Brigham and Women's Hospital, Harvard Medical School, 75 Francis Street, Boston, MA 02115, USA
* Corresponding author.
E-mail address: cdowney@llu.edu

to improve the quality of health care. One of the ways the ACA sought to achieve these goals was to tie physician and hospital reimbursements to delivery of quality care, rather than fee for service reimbursement. Quality care was translated into "value-based" delivery, and this aspect was so crucial for the success of the legislation overall that the Centers for Medicare and Medicaid Services introduced a new branch called the Centers for Medicare and Medicaid Innovation to help improve the value of care delivered in the United States.[1]

As a country, the United States spends more money providing worse outcomes than other similar countries.[2,3] The case for improving outcomes and reigning in costs on a national level is easy to make, but how should this impact medical training? Approximately 20% of all hospitals in the United States are teaching hospitals, where residents or fellows are providing at least a portion of the care administered. It would stand to reason that the quality of care delivered by the trainees at these sites contributes significantly to the overall quality of care provided.[4] The Accreditation Council for Graduate Medical Education (ACGME) provides guidance on specific milestones that each internal medicine subspecialty fellow, including rheumatology fellows, should have mastered before independent practice. Of these 24 currently published ACGME rheumatology subspecialty milestones, 7 of them directly relate to QI and practice improvement (**Table 1**).[5]

As the focus in care delivery shifts further and further toward increasing value for patients, so too should medical education.[6] Improving care delivery is a moving target and the process requires constant evaluation of the status quo. Because fellows must evaluate and reflect on the quality of care they provide, it is incumbent on faculty educators to both serve as role models and instructors with regard to best practices for life-long orientation toward QI.

One can argue the best way is to learn by doing, and several rheumatology fellow projects have not only made positive impacts on patient care, but also facilitated the learning of the fellow. To successfully teach QI in the rheumatology training environment, collaboration and innovation need to be fostered. This style of teaching requires knowledgeable, organized instructors working in a participatory setting toward the common goal of positive change to the system on varying levels. The goal of this review is to highlight the positive role fellows play in QI, explore the challenges associated with teaching QI to fellows and share existing QI resources for faculty and fellows. Although role modeling is a beneficial tool for teaching the QI process to trainees, there is value in formalizing a fellow-centric curriculum in this arena.

FELLOWS ROLE IN QUALITY IMPROVEMENT

Fellowship programs have a duty to their trainees to help them become proficient in the ACGME recommended milestones, however there is a case to be made for involving fellows in QI projects that transcends fulfilling training obligations. Rheumatology fellows are poised to make large impacts on the organizations they are a part of. Two of the Healthcare Effectiveness Data and Information Set (HEDIS) measures reported to the National Committee for Quality Assurance are directly related to rheumatological care: disease-modifying antirheumatic drug therapy for rheumatoid arthritis and osteoporosis testing and management in women older than 64. The HEDIS measures are indirectly tied to participation in health insurance networks, meaning the influence fellows can exert in these arenas can not only improve individual health but also result in financial benefits for their organizations.

The first step in any QI project is to assess the processes currently in place.[7] Residents and fellows are newcomers to the system and with fresh eyes can often spot

Table 1
Accreditation Council for Graduate Medical Education milestones for training

Milestone	Ready for Unsupervised Practice Relevant Behaviors	Aspirational Relevant Behaviors
Scholarship (MK3)	Collaborates with other investigators to design and complete a project related to clinical practice, quality improvement, patient safety, education, or research	Leads a scholarly project advancing clinical practice, quality improvement, patient safety, education, or research Publishes peer-reviewed article(s) containing scholarly work (clinical practice, quality improvement, patient safety, education, or research)
Works effectively within an interprofessional team (eg, with peers, consultants, nursing, ancillary professionals, and other support personnel). (SBP1)	Understands the roles and responsibilities of, and effectively partners with, all members of the team Efficiently coordinates activities of other team members to optimize care	Develops, trains, and inspires the team regarding unexpected events or new patient management strategies Viewed by other team members as a leader in the delivery of high-quality care
Recognizes system error and advocates for system improvement. (SBP2)	Identifies systemic causes of medical error and navigates them to provide safe patient care Advocates for safe patient care and optimal patient care systems Activates formal system resources to investigate and mitigate real or potential medical error Reflects on and learns from own critical incidents that may lead to medical error	Advocates for system leadership to formally engage in quality assurance and quality improvement activities Viewed as a leader in identifying and advocating for the prevention of medical error Teaches others regarding the importance of recognizing and mitigating system error
Identifies forces that impact the cost of health care, and advocates for and practices cost-effective care. (SBP3)	Consistently works to address patient-specific barriers to cost-effective care Advocates for cost conscious utilization of resources such as emergency department visits and hospital readmissions Incorporates cost awareness principles into standard clinical judgments and decision making, including use of screening tests	Teaches patients and health care team members to recognize and address common barriers to cost-effective care and appropriate utilization of resources Actively participates in initiatives and care delivery models designed to overcome or mitigate barriers to cost-effective, high-quality care
Monitors practice with a goal for improvement. (PBLI1)	Regularly self-reflects on one's practice or performance, and consistently acts on those reflections to improve practice Recognizes suboptimal practice or performance as an opportunity for learning and self-improvement	Regularly seeks external validation regarding self-reflection to maximize practice improvement Actively and independently engages in self-improvement efforts and reflects on the experience

(continued on next page)

Table 1
(continued)

Milestone	Ready for Unsupervised Practice Relevant Behaviors	Aspirational Relevant Behaviors
Learns and improves via performance audit. (PBLI2)	Analyzes own clinical performance data and actively works to improve performance Actively engages in opportunities to achieve focused education and performance improvement Demonstrates the ability to apply common principles and techniques of quality improvement to improve care for a panel of patients	Actively monitors clinical performance through various data sources Able to lead projects aimed at education and performance improvement Uses common principles and techniques of quality improvement to continuously improve care for a panel of patients
Learns and improves at the point of care. (PBLI4)	Routinely reconsiders an approach to a problem, asks for help, or seeks new information Routinely translates new medical information needs into well-formed clinical questions Guided by the characteristics of clinical questions, efficiently searches medical information resources, including decision support tools and guidelines Independently appraises clinical research reports based on accepted criteria	Role models how to appraise clinical research reports based on accepted criteria Has a systematic approach to track and pursue emerging clinical questions

Adapted from The Internal Medicine Subspecialty Milestones Project: A Joint Initiative of The Accreditation Council for Graduate Medical Education and The American Board of Internal Medicine. Available at https://www.acgme.org/Portals/0/PDFs/Milestones/InternalMedicineSubspecialtyMilestones.pdf?ver=2015-11-06-120527-673. Accessed Dec 20 2018; with permission.

problems the faculty may miss. They may bring with them previous experiences and a new perspective, enhancing their ability to see opportunities for change more than someone who has been in the system for a longer period of time. Conscious use of a trainee's indigenous learning provides an opportunity to enhance formal learning.

In addition to the potential gains to the organization as a whole, involving fellows in the process of QI allows overburdened faculty members to institute changes that they themselves may not have the bandwidth to enact themselves. Reporting on the findings leads to publications for the department and the faculty in addition to the obvious scholarly gains for the resident or fellow himself or herself. Although it is becoming more of the norm for medical students to learn about care delivery and process improvement during their didactic years in medical school, fellows and residents learn more from the culture of an institution than the lectures they receive while in training programs. Medicine is mostly learned at the bedside through patient interactions. The teaching of QI follows the same paradigm. Formal teaching is helpful, but it is only one step in a long process of education that is best acquired through planning, conducting, analyzing, and presenting their project first-hand. However, tacit learning in the setting of QI may not be optimal in all settings and care should be taken to uncover unconscious biases.

INVOLVING FELLOWS IN QUALITY IMPROVEMENT PROCESSES

Organizational learning, arguably the purpose of QI, occurs when individuals learn. Organizational learning processes involves teams who rely on global dialogue where they are free to engage in inquiry and collaboration. Collaboration in a nonpunitive environment may serve as the initial step into the QI plan-do-study-act cycle (PDSA cycle).[8] Brainstorming sessions can be an effective first step in implementation of PDSA.[9] Holding quarterly brainstorming sessions can allow for free flow of ideas and potentially lead to identification of patient safety or care delivery opportunities.

However, for trainees to feel the freedom to speak up about a problem and collaborate toward a solution, the culture of the department/division needs to be one wherein a trainee is not afraid to voice concerns about processes that are in place which may not be optimal. Fellows should be free to engage in inquiry and dialogue. In other words, psychological safety for trainees needs to be in place before they can be expected to experiment with new processes.[10] Creating this environment requires openness across boundaries, resilience and adaptability, and a culture that rewards innovation. Ultimately it is a process for creating shared meaning.

Role modeling is one way that newly minted physicians learn skills necessary to be an effective physician beyond direct patient care, such as professionalism.[11] Partnering a rheumatology fellow with a faculty advisor can allow for role modeling of the QI process and allow the fellow to work through a given problem with mentorship. Developing competence in practice improvement is skills-based and should be taught as such.[12]

For QI to take place, there needs to be a culture of psychological safety for the learners as well as a "change mentality" in the individual faculty members.[13] The health care organization overall, but more importantly rheumatology divisions themselves, should strive to foster environments that prioritize a focus on identifying ways care delivery can be improved. The hierarchical pedagogy must be replaced with a collaborative environment, and fellows need to be seen as equally important in the development of innovation as the faculty. This degree of systems-level thinking can be invoked when the very hegemony of the medical hierarchy is upended in the QI space, allowing for emancipatory thinking. This radical shift in the power structure creates space for new perspectives in process improvement and prevents perpetuation of the status quo.[14]

For a fellow to feel like he or she can speak up and advocate for change, the culture of the organization should convey inclusiveness. Leader inclusiveness is positively associated with psychological safety, which predicts engagement in QI work.[15] The culture of the rheumatology program should focus on connection and relationships where fellows can see themselves as constructors of knowledge. Thus, the power dynamic is shifted from attending physician as ruler to one where the duty and privilege of power is shared.[16] In the end everyone benefits, the teachers, the learners, the organization, and especially the patient.[17]

LEARNING COLLABORATIVES AND FORMAL CURRICULA

Although there are 39 academic institutions around the world that have developed a formal curriculum for residents using the Institute for Healthcare Improvement (IHI) Open School for Graduate Medical Education, most of which require completion to finish residency, there are no rheumatology fellowship programs that have created such teaching models.[18]

Such learning collaboration is one way to further create a change culture in fellowship teaching curriculum. One design that the IHI Open School for Graduate Medical Education has developed to aid in the teaching and implementation of quality care delivery is the Breakthrough Series Learning Collaborative.[19] The mission of the learning collaborative is to allow organizations to learn best practices from each other to improve current health care delivery.

Learning Collaboratives can serve to fill gaps in knowledge or expertise. This can deepen fellow understanding of identification of system error and effecting change by linking fellows to experts not available locally. One such learning collaborative that successfully engages pediatric rheumatology trainees is the Pediatric Rheumatology Care and Outcomes Improvement Network (PR-COIN). PR-COIN serves as a model for teaching improvement and implementation science to fellows in locations where faculty expertise may not be readily available.

Although there is arguably a dearth of formal settings for teaching rheumatology fellows the essentials of QI practices, the University of California, San Francisco (UCSF) created an innovative program in 2012 that involved rheumatology fellows directly. Although in this instance the fellows were the teachers and not the learners, a useful tool in adult learning. Reallocation of perspective and positionality allows fellows new perspective and authority, thus permitting authority of voice which may have been suppressed if they were in a position of lower power.[20]

This year-long experimental training course was started in the UCSF Action Research Program as a course in implementation science. Rheumatology fellows aided by faculty oversaw 4 first-year medical students in a year-long process of hands-on learning about QI. All 4 first-year medical students completed an individual QI project with the assistance of the rheumatology fellows and faculty.

The projects completed by these medical students included FRAX tool integration into the electronic health record, improving no-show rates, and creating a health coaching intervention to improve patient understanding of high-risk medication understanding.[21] To expand on this project, and reinforce the concept of QI as a process rather than an end, it would have been fruitful for the first-year medical students to return to the rheumatology clinic as fourth-year medical students to see if their processes had stood the test of time. Investigating the challenges their projects have faced in continuity over the intervening 3 years would further showcase first-hand the challenges in process improvement. To make a project such as this one successful, the faculty must be given adequate time in his or her schedule to properly mentor not only the fellows involved, but the medical students as well.

CHALLENGES OF TEACHING QUALITY IMPROVEMENT TO FELLOWS

Among trainees, QI projects are uniquely popular. Most rheumatology fellowships span just 2 years, and many fellows will agree that trying to learn the entirety of the specialty in that time is an onerous if not impossible task. The demands on a trainee's attention outside of medical knowledge acquisition are numerous and time for conducting research in the fellows' schedule is scarce. The PDSA cycle is meant to be repeated early and often, making completion of an initiative with sharable data possible in an academic term for fellows.[12]

One challenge with QI projects is that QI is a process, not an end point. Unless there is a faculty champion that can extend the life of the process beyond the tenure of the particular fellow with the organization, the process likely reverts to the structure in place before the initiation of the new process. For learning to be transformational, there must be a mechanism to capture, nurture and disseminate a new vision. There is a lack of data showing the long-term outcomes of fellow initiated projects.

Another challenge with teaching QI is the comfort level of the faculty with this arena. For faculty not familiar with QI themselves, arguably the best resource for helping faculty members teach QI to their trainees is the IHI Open School. Included with the cost of a subscription to the Web site, the IHI graduate medical education (GME) faculty course series includes training in the reasoning behind including trainees in the process, the role of the faculty member, the role of didactics, aligning GME education and organization goals, and provides a roadmap for facilitating projects.[22] For no charge, a fellow project can be submitted to the IHI Open School for critique, a resource to help both the mentor and mentee improve on his or her skills.

The nature of being a fellow may in itself be a challenge to performing and thus learning the QI process. The transitional nature of fellowship training may decrease the fellow's sense of agency in effective change. As the fellow is moving toward a level of higher responsibility in patient care, the perceived risk of recognizing system error is also increased.[23]

Rheumatology Trainee Quality Improvement Projects

The value of formal didactic teaching should not be underestimated. However, the medical pedagogy is continually evolving to use more "learn by doing" techniques of teaching and is rooted in "see one, do one, teach one." Many rheumatology fellows learn to implement QI processes by completing one from start to finish, and many faculty members learn to teach QI by mentoring and overseeing a fellow project from the ground up. These projects can be a boon to the faculty mentor as he or she can increase his or her academic publication footprint when copublishing with and mentoring a fellow. It is difficult to quantify how many fellow projects go on to be published and even harder to quantify what happens to these projects once the fellows have left their institutions. The following are several examples of fellow projects that showcase the learn by doing approach and have led to better patient outcomes.

Collaboration leading to improved patient and organization outcomes: optimization of nurse visits and encounters

Second-year fellow, Dr Shazdeh Butt, at Geisinger Medical Center along with her mentor Dr Eric Newman, incorporated their system's unique needs and resources to cut back on unnecessary follow-up visits for stable patients. A nurse-only telephone visit replaced in-office visits for stable patients. The nurse was trained to ask a series of questions that would indicate the patient needed to be seen in clinic and reviewed the laboratory results for medication monitoring. The intervention was found on average to save patients $54 in appointment-associated costs and 2 hours and 10 minutes of traveling to and from the appointment. Patients were also highly satisfied with the outcome of the nurse visit when compared with physically seeing the physician for a routine quarterly check in. The nurse only telephone encounter further improved access for sick patients who needed to be seen in the clinic.[24] By improving the availability of clinic visits for higher level of care patients, the increased billing levels improved the overall income to the system as well. "This was a highly successful and sustained project, as everyone benefited. The patient benefited by saving time and money when they were otherwise doing fine; the provider team and system benefited by improving access for patients that were not doing well. The nurses enjoyed interacting with the patients by phone. The IT lift was minimal, and the program has been sustained for over 4 years." Eric Newman, Geisinger Medical Center.

The intervention was created and designed by mentor faculty Dr Newman and implemented by second-year fellow Dr Butt. This project demonstrates an instance in which fellow and faculty collaboration led to identification of a need that was unique to the training environment and development of an innovative work-around in care delivery. The project maintained patient safety by training nurses to monitor for abnormal laboratory values and red-flags in the patient phone interview. Eliminating the in-person visit drove patient satisfaction and was able to improve overall access to care by conserving a scare resource: the outpatient rheumatology clinic slot.

The environment at Geisinger nurtured the psychological safety that allowed this fellow/faculty pair to create an innovative change in the usual care delivery and the freedom to implement such a radical shift by using faculty collaboration to engage in cooperative problem solving. This type of project also relies on a change culture that is not afraid to veer from the status quo and adopt a hypothesis testing approach to daily operations. The resources at Geisinger needed to be allocated to allow for the nursing staff to be properly trained. The division culture also had to extend to the member of the nursing staff making the calls. He or she had a to be willing to change his or her duties. Further, the division had to be willing to divert the duties of the phone nurse away from other tasks to making telephone encounters.

Improving patient outcomes: pneumococcal vaccination

More importantly than helping the organization and the department/division, fellow involvement in QI projects translates to better care delivery for the patient. A particularly fruitful area for fellows looking to practice their QI skills is in vaccination rate improvement. Every year there are at least 3 fellow abstracts accepted to the American College of Rheumatology Annual Meeting centered on improving pneumococcal vaccination rates alone. Loyola University Fellow Melissa Bussey successfully completed one such pneumococcal vaccination project in 2014. Through her intervention, the rate of vaccine-eligible patients younger than 65 was more than tripled. For those patients older than 65, the rates of vaccination were almost doubled.[25] Similar results were achieved at the University of California-San Francisco by then fellow Alison Bays. This rheumatology fellow project lead to an improvement in pneumococcal vaccination rates from 12% to 52% in just 10 months.[26]

Improvement projects such as these involving immunization rates make for optimal teaching examples and initiations into the world of QI processes for many reasons. First, there are clear requirements and recommendations about who should be vaccinated and when. Second, immunizations tend to be an area that always have room for improvement as rates tend to drop when there is no concerted effort by the providers to administer the immunizations.[27] Further, there are clear and measurable outcomes: vaccinated, nor not vaccinated. The data are easily obtained from the electronic health record and the data are often easy to manipulate without the help of a hired statistician. They also tend to be successful, empowering the trainee to then attempt to effect change in other areas of care delivery. Last, these projects inarguably improve the care of the patients at these centers as it has been well established that pneumococcal vaccinations prevent illness, hospitalizations and death.[28]

Addressing an unmet need: osteoporosis documentation

At University of Texas, Southwestern Medical Center, second-year fellow Brittany Ahmed designed an electronic health record prompt alerting fellows and rotating residents to improve documentation of osteoporosis in veterans with rheumatoid arthritis, leading to significant increase in documentation. Improving the documentation of bone health in this population naturally leads to higher rates of addressing the problem at the individual patient level. Implementation of this prompt successfully increased the rate of dual-energy x-ray absorptiometry documentation from 58% to an average of 76% over a 3-month period.[29] Further work needs to be done to determine if increased documentation of bone health actually led to an increase in prescriptions written for osteoporosis treatment.

This project, like many others, are examples of the collaboration and resources that are necessary for fellows to undertake QI at their respective institutions. The fellow who recognizes the opportunity for improved processes must establish buy-in from a faculty mentor to sponsor the project within the institution. As many projects often translate to changes in the electronic health delivery systems, buy-in must also be sought from the technological support departments. As anyone with experience at a large system can attest, changing the electronic health system (EHS) is far from nimble. In many institutions, approval and implementation in changes to the EHS often takes weeks to months. Depending on the changes sought and the software involved, updating the EHS can also be costly and fellow QI projects may not have the financial resources to make the changes to the electronic health system.

Improving fellow care delivery: outcome measures in rheumatoid arthritis

In addition to improving care delivery at the level of the system, fellow QI projects can also serve to help teach fellows about their own patient care and how to improve it.[30] An example is a project done by third-year Brigham and Women's Hospital rheumatology fellow Dr Cianna Leatherwood.[31] Her project's goal was to incorporate patient reported outcomes into a treat to target approach for rheumatoid arthritis. The team at Brigham and Women's Hospital worked to capture Routine Assessment of Patient Index Data 3 (RAPID3) measures on iPads completed by patients in the waiting room. The intervention group lead to a higher percentage of patients with rheumatoid arthritis getting to their treatment target than the control group, thus improving disease control and patient outcomes in this population. This project's innovation comes from the presence of iPads in the patient waiting room, which can be a costly intervention if the technology is not already in place at an institution.

This project is an excellent example of transformative learning for rheumatology fellow Dr Leatherwood. She was able to use her QI project as a springboard to learn more about validated patient questionnaires and treat to target philosophy. These types of projects force fellows to reflect about their current practices. Part of this fellow's intervention was to involve her faculty in a learning collaborative about treat to target in rheumatoid arthritis using RAPID3 as a measure of success. Witnessing faculty change their behavior based on a fellow intervention contributes to the culture of humble inquiry and the notion that even the masters in the field can always have room for improvement.[32] The fellow had the opportunity to experience her superiors undergo transformations in how they practice medicine based on her implementation of patient data, a powerful reminder that each of us should be striving to improve. Having a culture in which the faculty walk the walk and engage in these projects does more to project the value of these projects than any formal teaching a faculty member can give a rheumatology fellow.

Involving fellow learning daily: fracture liaison service

Fracture Liaison Services (FLS) are an informal way for fellows to experience the value and efficacy of QI without the formalized structure of developing de novo processes. Loma Linda University Medical Center is one institution that has developed an FLS in which the fellows take active part. This is an organic opportunity for fellows to analyze a process that is already in place and find ways to improve on it, thus improving patient care. One such fellow, Donna Jose of Loma Linda University, found that most patients who were evaluated by the FLS went on to out-of-network primary care physicians.[33] Those patients were lost to follow-up and data are not available about their rates of pharmacologic intervention. She posed that hiring a coordinator to ensure a more seamless transition from the inpatient to outpatient settings would improve the post-fracture treatment rate by ensuring that patients were seen by someone with expertise in osteoporosis.

SUMMARY

Rheumatology fellows in training can and should be included in projects that aim to improve the value of care delivery. Active collaborative participation in QI projects allows faculty to evaluate the fellow's competence in at least 7 domains laid out in the ACGME guidelines for independent rheumatology practice. Even more importantly, fellow-driven projects can improve the care their patients receive. There are unique challenges in championing rheumatology fellow QI projects, such a lack of expertise or experience among faculty members, scarcity of formal teaching curricula, and potentially the division's attitudes toward change and innovation. However, these challenges can be overcome through experience. After all, trial and error is the very nature of the QI process. To be comfortable with the ambiguity of doing something for the first time, the division must implement a safe learning environment that encourages a growth mindset. Other investigators have made the link between psychological safety and the willingness to participate in QI.[15] Creating a culture of mutual respect among faculty and fellows has cascading effects and can improve the effectiveness of the faculty and fellows' willingness to advocate for system change and ultimately better patient care,[34] which is the driving force behind everything we do as physicians.

REFERENCES

1. Home page, Center for Medicare & Medicaid Innovation. Available at: https://innovation.cms.gov. Accessed December 23, 2018.

2. Sawyer B, Gonzales S. How does the quality of the U. S. healthcare system compare to other countries? Kaiser Family Foundation. Available at: https://www.healthsystemtracker.org/chart-collection/quality-u-s-healthcare-system-compare-countries/. Accessed December 25, 2018.

3. Sawyer B, Cox C. How does health spending in the U.S. compare to other countries? Kaiser Family Foundation. Available at: https://www.healthsystemtracker.org/chart-collection/health-spending-u-s-compare-countries/#item-relative-size-wealth-u-s-spends-disproportionate-amount-health. Accessed December 25, 2018.

4. Young JQ, Ranji SR, Wachter RM, et al. "July effect": impact of the academic year-end changeover on patient outcomes: a systematic review. Ann Intern Med 2011;155:309–15.

5. The Internal Medicine Subspecialty Milestones Project, a joint initiative of the accreditation council for graduate medical education and the American Board of Internal Medicine. Available at: https://www.acgme.org/Portals/0/PDFs/Milestones/InternalMedicineSubspecialtyMilestones.pdf?ver=2015-11-06-120527-673. Accessed December 20, 2018.

6. Porter ME, Teisberg EO. Redefining health care: creating value-based competition on results. Boston: Harvard Business School Press; 2006.

7. Langley GJ, Nolan KM, Nolan TW, et al. The improvement guide: a practical approach to enhancing organizational performance. San Francisco: Jossey-Bass Publishers; 1996.
8. Leis JA, Shojania KG. A primer on PDSA: executing plan–do–study–act cycles in practice, not just in name. BMJ Qual Saf 2017;26:572–7.
9. van Bokhoven MA, Kok G, van der Weijden T. Designing a quality improvement intervention: a systematic approach. BMJ Qual Saf 2003;12:215–20.
10. Nembhard I, Edmondson A. Psychological safety: a foundation for speaking up, collaboration, and experimentation in organizations. In: The oxford handbook of positive organizational scholarship. Oxford University Press; 2011. Available at: http://www.oxfordhandbooks.com/view/10.1093/oxfordhb/9780199734610.001.0001/oxfordhb-9780199734610-e-037. Accessed March 2, 2019.
11. Johnston S. See one, do one, teach one: developing professionalism across generations. Clin Orthop Relat Res 2006;449:186–92.
12. Ogrinc G, Headrick LA, Mutha S, et al. A framework for teaching medical students and residents about practice-based learning and improvement, synthesized from a literature review. Acad Med 2003;78(7):748–56.
13. Wong BM, Levinson W, Shojania KG. Quality improvement in medical education: current state and future directions. Med Educ 2012;46:107–19.
14. Hooks B. Teaching to transgress. New York: Rutledge; 1994.
15. Nembhard IM, Edmondson AC. Making it safe: the effects of leader inclusiveness and professional status on psychological safety and improvement efforts in health care teams. J Organ Behav 2006;27:941–66.
16. Tisdell E. Poststructural feminist pedagogies: the possibilities and limitations of feminist emancapatory adult learning theory and practice. Adult Educ Q 1998; 48(10):139–56.
17. Edmondson AC. Learning from mistakes is easier said than done: Group and organizational influences on the detection and correction of human error. J Appl Behav Sci 2004;40(1):66–90.
18. Academic organizations using the IHI open school online courses. Available at: http://www.ihi.org/education/IHIOpenSchool/Courses/Documents/CurriculumList Academic.pdf. Accessed December 23, 2018.
19. The Breakthrough series: IHI's collaborative model for achieving Breakthrough improvement. IHI innovation series white paper. Boston: Institute for Healthcare Improvement; 2003. Available at: www.IHI.org.
20. Middleton S. A postmodern pedagogy for the sociology of women's education. In: Arnot M, Weiler K. Feminism and social justice in education: international perspectives. London: Falmer Press. p. 39–70.
21. Goglin S, Margaretten M, Trupin L, et al. New frontiers: teaching quality improvement to first year medical students in a rheumatology safety net clinic:abstract. Arthritis Rheumatol 2015;67(suppl 10). Available at: https://acrabstracts.org/abstract/new-frontiers-teaching-quality-improvement-to-first-year-medical-students-in-a-rheumatology-safety-net-clinic/. Accessed December 25, 2018.
22. IHI Open School GME Faculty Training Courses. Available at: http://www.ihi.org/education/IHIOpenSchool/Chapters/Groups/Faculty/Pages/Courses.aspx. Accessed December 23, 2018.
23. Torralba KD, Loo LK, Byrne JM, et al. Does psychological safety impact the clinical learning environment for resident physicians? Results from the VA's learners' perceptions survey. J Grad Med Educ 2016;8(5):699–707.
24. Butt S, Newman E, Smith N. Nurse scheduled telephone visit: the right rheumatology care for the right patient at the right time: abstract. Arthritis Rheumatol 2016;68(suppl

10). Available at: https://acrabstracts.org/abstract/nurse-scheduled-telephone-visit-the-right-rheumatology-care-for-the-right-patient-at-the-right-time/. Accessed December 25, 2018.

25. Bussey M, Ostrowski AO. A quality improvement initiative to improve pneumococcal vaccination rates in immunosuppressed patient: abstract. Arthritis Rheumatol 2014. ACR/ARHP Annual Meeting. Available at: https://acrabstracts.org/abstract/a-quality-improvement-initiative-to-improve-pneumococcal-vaccination-rates-in-immunosuppressed-patients/. Accessed December 24, 2018.

26. Bays A, Nayak RR, Murray S, et al. Improving pneumococcal vaccination rates for immunosuppressed patients in an academic rheumatology clinic [abstract]. Arthritis Rheumatol 2016;68(suppl 10). Available at: https://acrabstracts.org/abstract/improving-pneumococcal-vaccination-rates-for-immunosuppressed-patients-in-an-academic-rheumatology-clinic/. Accessed December 27, 2018.

27. Williams WW, Lu P-J, O'Halloran A, et al. Noninfluenza vaccination coverage among adults—United States, 2012. MMWR Morb Mortal Wkly Rep 2014;63: 95–102.

28. Centers for Disease Control and Prevention. In: Hamborsky J, Kroger A, Wolfe S, editors. Epidemiology and prevention of vaccine-preventable diseases. 13th edition. Washington (DC): Public Health Foundation; 2015.

29. Ahmed B, Nayfe R, Udupa A, et al. Documenting bone health for veterans with rheumatoid arthritis in an outpatient academic clinic: abstract. Arthritis Rheumatol 2018;70(suppl 10). Available at: https://acrabstracts.org/abstract/documenting-bone-health-for-veterans-with-rheumatoid-arthritis-in-an-outpatient-academic-clinic/. Accessed December 25, 2018.

30. Wong BM, Etchells EE, Kuper A, et al. Teaching quality improvement and patient safety to trainees, a systemic review. Acad Med 2010;85(9):1425–39.

31. Forman M, Leatherwood C, Xu C, et al. Implementation of a treat-to-target quality improvement program for rheumatoid arthritis management using real-time patient reported outcome measures:abstract. Arthritis Rheumatol 2018;70(suppl 10). Available at: https://acrabstracts.org/abstract/implementation-of-a-treat-to-target-quality-improvement-program-for-rheumatoid-arthritis-management-using-real-time-patient-reported-outcome-measures/. Accessed December 24, 2018.

32. Houchens N, Harrod M, Moody S, et al. Techniques and behaviors associated with exemplary inpatient general medicine teaching: an exploratory qualitative study. J Hosp Med 2017;7:503–9.

33. Jose D, Torralba K, Downey C, et al. Fracture liaison service in an open health system: outcomes and challenges. In: Arthritis & rheumatology, vol. 70. Hoboken (NJ): WILEY; 2018.

34. Domen RE. The ethics of ambiguity: rethinking the role and importance of uncertainty in medical education and practice. Acad Pathol 2016;3. 2374289516654712.

Underserved Communities
Enhancing Care with Graduate Medical Education

Vaneet K. Sandhu, MD[a],*, Donna M. Jose, MD[b],
Candace H. Feldman, MD, MPH, ScD[c]

KEYWORDS

- Population health • Health services • Graduate medical education • Underserved
- Health disparities

KEY POINTS

- The disproportionate decrease in supply of rheumatology providers to anticipated demand in the coming years warrants a change in the education system.
- Health equity is limited by disparities in life expectancy, quality of life, rates of morbidity and mortality, disease severity, and access to health care.
- Expanding medical training to medically underserved areas increases the likelihood of physician retention in primary and subspecialty care in these areas.
- Using technologies to expand on health care access as well as medical education is a rapidly emerging field of health care.
- Formal health disparities teaching in medical education curriculum will provide an environment dedicated to service learning in a community-based approach, benefiting patients and learners alike.

The American Medical Association recently released a statement defining health equity as "optimal health for all," and affirming the organization's commitment to promote better health care access, diversity in the health care workforce, understanding of the social determinants of health, and equitable distribution of resources and high-quality care.[1] Unfortunately, according to a World Health Organization report in 2015, approximately 400 million individuals globally lack access to at least 1 of 7 essential health services as a result of workforce shortages and uneven distributions of health

[a] Department of Internal Medicine, Division of Rheumatology, Loma Linda University, Loma Linda University Medical Center, 11234 Anderson Street, Suite 1521, Loma Linda, CA 92354, USA; [b] Department of Internal Medicine, Loma Linda University, 11234 Anderson Street, Loma Linda, CA 92354, USA; [c] Department of Medicine, Division of Rheumatology, Inflammation and Immunity, Brigham and Women's Hospital, 60 Fenwood Road, Office 6016P, Boston, MA 02115, USA
* Corresponding author.
E-mail address: vksandhu@llu.edu

Rheum Dis Clin N Am 46 (2020) 167–178
https://doi.org/10.1016/j.rdc.2019.09.009
0889-857X/20/© 2019 Elsevier Inc. All rights reserved.

care workers.[2] In a statement published in 2001, the Institute of Medicine declared that "All health care organizations, professional groups, and private and public purchasers should adopt as their explicit purpose to continually reduce the burden of illness, injury, and disability, and to improve the health and functioning of the people of the United States."[3]

RURAL AMERICA

One in 5 individuals living in the United States resides in a rural area.[4] **Fig. 1** depicts the distribution across the United States of urban clusters, defined by a population of 2500 to fewer than 50,000 people, and urbanized clusters, defined by a population in excess of 50,000 people.[5] In 2010, of approximately 4000 rheumatologists practicing in the United States, 90% were in metropolitan regions (labor market areas centered on an urbanized cluster), 3% in micropolitan (labor market areas centered on an urban cluster), and 7% in rural parts of the United States.[5,6] In urban clusters, many patients travel in excess of 100 miles to see a rheumatologist.[6] Interestingly, despite the declining rural population and pullulating urban population, and despite the greater density of physicians in more populous regions, the physician-to-patient ratio remains disparate and inadequate.

In 2015, the American College of Rheumatology Workforce Study iterated that the percentage of internal medicine residents entering rheumatology has remained stable at approximately 4% from 2005 to 2015.[7,8] With a retiring baby-boomer population of physicians, the challenge is the estimated disproportionate decrease of supply

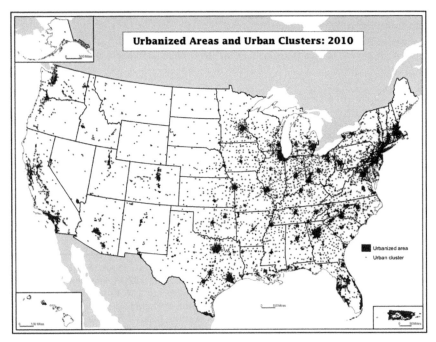

Fig. 1. Urbanized areas and urban clusters, defined by population of 50,000 or more and 2500 to less than 50,000, respectively. U.S. Census Bureau, 2010 Census Urban Area Delineation Program. (*From* United States Census Bureau. Urbanized Areas and Urban Clusters: 2010. Available at: https://www.census.gov/library/visualizations/2010/geo/ua2010_uas_and_ucs_map.html. Accessed Jan 28 2019.)

compared with demand for rheumatology services. With a baseline clinical full-time equivalent (FTE) of 4997 in 2015, the 2025 projected supply will decrease by 27% to 3645 FTE and the 2030 projected supply will further decrease by 30% from baseline to 3455 FTE (**Fig. 2**).[8] There is also a significant shortage of pediatric rheumatologists. For the nearly 300,000 children with arthritis in the United States,[9] we have fewer than 350 board-certified and practicing pediatric rheumatologists, 8 states without a single board-certified and practicing pediatric rheumatologist, and 4 states with only 1.[10] Interestingly, there is a significantly higher concentration of adult rheumatology training programs in the Northeast and mid-Atlantic regions compared with areas west of the Mississippi (with the exception of California, **Fig. 3**). These findings are in line with a study published by the American Association of Medical Colleges in early 2018 stating the projected shortage of physicians in the United States of approximately 43,000 to 121,000 by 2030.[11] This same study demonstrated that, if individuals living in non-metropolitan areas and those without insurance used health care in the same way as those insured individuals living in metropolitan areas, the United States would have needed more than 30,000 additional physicians. Although this may certainly represent, to some degree, overuse of the health care system in urban areas, there is no question of limited access to quality health care in rural areas. The Health Resources and Services Administration designates "medically underserved areas" (MUAs) as areas with a shortage of primary care health services, high infant mortality, high poverty or a high elderly population,[12] and Health Professional Shortage Areas (HPSAs), as geographic areas, facilities, or populations with shortages of primary medical care, dental, or mental health providers,[12] and highlights the need for increased resource allocation in these areas. What is, however, less discussed, is the value and importance of medical education in these underserved areas.

THE RESPONSIBILITY OF HEALTH EQUITY: ADDRESSING WORKFORCE SHORTAGE

The National Center for Chronic Disease Prevention and Health Promotion states "Health equity is achieved when every person has the opportunity to 'attain his or

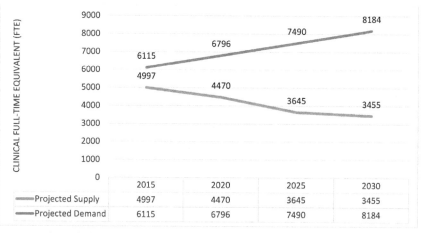

	2015	2020	2025	2030
Projected Supply	4997	4470	3645	3455
Projected Demand	6115	6796	7490	8184

Fig. 2. Supply and demand of adult rheumatologists in the United States (clinical FTE). (*Adapted from* Battafarano DF, Ditmyer M, Bolster MB, et al. 2015 American College of Rheumatology Workforce Study: Supply and Demand Projections of Adult Rheumatology Workforce, 2015-2030. Arthritis Care Res(Hoboken) 2018;70(4):623; with permission.)

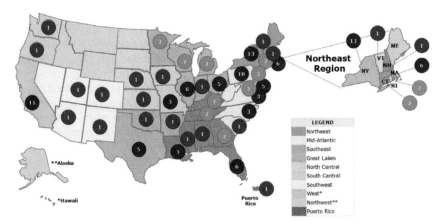

Fig. 3. Number of adult rheumatology training programs in each US state in 2015. (*From* Bolster MB, Bass AR, Hausmann JS, et al. 2015 American College of Rheumatology Workforce Study: The Role of Graduate Medical Education in Adult Rheumatology. Arthritis & Rheumatology 2018;70(6):821; with permission.)

her full potential' and no one is 'disadvantaged from achieving this potential because of social position or other socially determined circumstances.'"[13] Disparities in life expectancy, quality of life, rates of morbidity and mortality, disease severity, and access to care result in health inequities. To begin to address this, the Centers for Disease Control and Prevention established programs like REACH (Racial and Ethnic Approaches to Community Health), which funds culturally appropriate interventions to reduce preventable risk behaviors such as poor nutrition and smoking.[13]

Achieving health equity requires a proper understanding of the community context. In underserved communities in particular it is important to appreciate the regional needs to provide high-quality health care. It is in part the responsibility of health professional schools to train high-quality health care providers in underserved regions. Ferguson and colleagues[14] and Ko and colleagues[15] demonstrated that a student's training, including their medical education experience, bears a large impact on the student's intention to practice in an MUA.

Medical Training: Expanding to Medically Underserved Areas

Increasing residency and fellowship positions, as well as salary support through grant programs will certainly help with the physician shortage crisis we are experiencing. Federally Qualified Health Centers (FQHCs) are community-based organizations that provide primary and preventive care services typically to MUAs. Such FQHCs as the Social Action Community Health System (SACHS) in San Bernardino, California, also involve specialty services like rheumatology to improve access to health care. An additional benefit at SACHS includes provision of funding to support resident salaries.

In surveys sent to Massachusetts community health center physician medical directors, more than 50% of directors felt that their patients needed better access to rheumatologic care.[16] Most providers were uncomfortable starting a disease-modifying antirheumatic drug or immunosuppressive medication and language differences and insurance status were deemed as barriers to obtaining appropriate rheumatologic care.[16] Placing trainees, including residents and fellows, in MUAs and HPSAs would then increase the likelihood of physician retention in both primary and subspecialty care, as residents tend to practice close to where they train.[17] One such example of integrating trainees into community health care includes training at the Riverside University Health System (RUHS), a community-based hospital whose rheumatology clinic is represented largely by a minority population. At RUHS, trainees are exposed to challenges ranging from complicated rheumatic manifestations (likely related to underutilization of health care services) to authorization for standard health care services and utilization of interpreter services. In addition, with regard to provider retention, I am an example of a trainee who returned to provide services at this facility.

Socioeconomic incentives will also improve physician likelihood of practicing in rural settings. This can be carried out by increased federal funding for programs such as the Conrad 30 Waiver Program, Title VII/VIII workforce development, the National Health Service Corps, and similar programs directed toward encouraging provision of health services to underserved communities, particularly places where shortages of subspecialists exist.

Telemedicine

An emerging field of health care, telemedicine provides an alternative approach to enhancing both physician education and patient access to health care with a focus on MUAs and HPSAs. Chase and colleagues[18,19] first reported the use of telemedicine in rheumatology at the Texas state prison where a remote-site examiner (physician on-site at the prison) was assigned as the "presenter." Although the study concluded that providers and prison staff were satisfied with the service and the consults were "equal" to on-site evaluation by a rheumatologist, critics note the concern with relying on proxy examinations by presenters with different levels of training.[20–22] An additional factor that comes into play is the cost of equipment needed for telemedicine presentation and transmission to a specialist. According to a systematic review by McDougall and colleagues[22] looking at 20 studies on the use of telemedicine in rheumatic diseases, most demonstrated cost-effectiveness but was noted that additional studies are warranted to justify its implementation for the diagnosis and management of rheumatic disease. In particular, diagnosing a new condition may require greater confidence in the physical examination, as well as identifying which rheumatic disease would most benefit from telemedicine services is warranted.[22]

Because of the scarcity of board-certified and practicing pediatric rheumatologists, telemedicine appears to be an excellent option for enhancing patient access. In a rural MUA in northern California, barriers in access to subspecialty care included traveling for more than 1 hour for appointments, missing work for appointments, and relying on emergency room visits.[23] Provision of telemedicine consultations on 55 children with special health care needs in this same area resulted in a high satisfaction with telemedicine in providing accessible, family-centered, and well-coordinated care with health care providers.[23] However, in a separate study evaluating patient barriers to accessing pediatric rheumatologic care, in-person visits were preferred by 95% over the option of telemedicine, even in cases in which travel to the pediatric rheumatology clinic exceeded 3 hours (28%).[24]

In telemedicine, an additional opportunity to be noted is for provider education. An example of this is Project Extension for Community Healthcare Outcomes, where primary care providers in local communities are linked with specialists from academic institutions who provide feedback and mentoring to provide high-quality care to patients with otherwise limited access to specialty services.[25] Through telemedicine and Internet-based tools, providers (nurse practitioners, primary care providers, physician assistants, pharmacists, and more) present patients through video- or telephone-conferencing in a patient-centered case-based format to university specialists. This method of patient care not only enhances the community-based provider's medical knowledge but also bears potential to affect feelings of professional stagnation and isolation with excess workloads and lack of access to consultation services; all recipes for accelerated burnout. In addition, this is a capacity-building approach and strengthens the skills and knowledge of existing providers rather than relying on external, visiting volunteers who may be less sustainable.

Another approach to using communication networks to improve patient access to health care services is electronic consultations: "e-consults." E-consults are "an asynchronous communication between health care providers that occurs within a shared electronic health record or secure Web-based platform."[26] Although not designed for routine chronic care, e-consults may be helpful in triaging consultations from referring providers to specialists, who may answer a clinical question, request additional information, and/or schedule a face-to-face appointment. It is important to note here that e-consults are not, with very few exceptions, official patient care encounters but are rather likened to "curbside consults." Loma Linda University Rheumatology partakes in e-consults through the Multi-County eConsult Initiative, serving Riverside and San Bernardino Counties in California. This system has opened a channel of communication between our local primary care providers and a rheumatologist that extends beyond direct patient-related tasks to also include some key education points, relayed electronically, on routine rheumatologic evaluation.

In addition to improving health care access, health care utilization services may be optimized by minimizing no-show rates, ensuring diagnostic testing is complete at the time of consultation services, and inclusion of learners in the e-consult experience will provide an avenue of medical learning that is likely to play a large role in health care in the coming years.

J-1 Visa Waiver Program

The J-1 visa waiver is a program typically handled by the US Department of Health and Human Services and/or the US Department of Veterans Affairs and is provided usually to individuals also known as international medical graduates (IMGs) who graduated from medical schools outside of the United States. Individuals carrying a J-1 visa are subject to a 2-year home-country physical presence requirement if they participated in a program to receive graduate medical education or training.[27] This requires a J-1 visa holder to return to his or her home country for a total of at least 2 years (cumulatively). Until this requirement is fulfilled, their J-1 visa status cannot be changed to an H-visa (nonimmigrant temporary worker) or intracompany transferee (L), nor can they receive an immigrant visa, a temporary worker (H), or fiancé (K) visa.[27] However, through the US Citizenship and Immigration Services, a waiver may be requested by a designated State Public Health Department (or its equivalent) in what is known as the Conrad State 30 Program, an opportunity limited to 30 waivers per department per federal fiscal year.[27] If a medical graduate (typically after completing training; ie, residency and/or fellowship) has an offer of full-time employment for 40 hours a week for at least 3 years and is willing to begin employment within 90 days of receiving a waver in a designated HPSA or a facility serving patients from such an area, he or she can apply for the Conrad State 30 Program.[27] Because more than 30% of rheumatology fellows in training are non-US medical school graduates,[28] increasing the number of J-1 waiver slots in MUAs, as well as providing better resources for renewing visas in these individuals, would likely help the ongoing shortage of rheumatologists. Alternatively, if IMGs elect to carry out their waiver in their home country for 2 years, they can come back to the United States and work under an H-1 work visa. Making this option more widely available can help prepare medical centers or clinics across the country anticipate their institution's needs, and plan for hiring such individuals back into the US rheumatology workforce. Doing a home country 2-year waiver might actually also be a better option for some IMGs, as the time to acquiring an H1 visa is much shorter (2 years) as compared with going through the Conrad State 30 Program.

The National Health Service Corps

The National Health Service Corps (NHSC) provides financial support through scholarships and loan repayment after graduation from some form of schooling for health professionals who provide primary care services in HPSAs.[29] More than 50,0000 health professionals have served in the NHSC since 1972 and, with nearly 11,000 current members, the NHSC provides services to more than 11 million people at more than 5000 urban, rural, and tribal sites. The program enables health professionals who might have personal financial limitations to deliver care in MUAs and HPSAs. Additional resources offered by the NHSC include funding for more than 1000 NHSC scholars who are currently either in school or residency.[29]

TRAINING BENEFITS IN UNDERSERVED AREAS

The Health Professional Schools in Service to the Nation Program was designed to reform medical education curriculum by defining service learning as "a structured learning experience that combines community service with explicit learning objectives, preparation and reflection," enabling students to "provide direct community service but also to learn about the context in which service is provided, the connection between their service and their academic coursework, and their roles as citizens."[30] Twenty institutions participated in this program from 1995 to 1998 through the Center for the Health Professions at the University of California at San Francisco. On evaluation at the second year of the program's commencement, service learning was deemed a powerful tool for influencing students in their outlook on the role of service in their lives as health care professionals.[31] In addition, community partners valued the ability to establish partnerships with academic institutions, particularly when their key role in shaping the education of these future health care professionals was recognized.[31] Socially accountable health professional education programs are along this spectrum of service learning designed to connect medical education curriculum with research and service that is unique to the needs of the population they serve.[32,33] It is through this community-based medical education that students are immersed within the community of their medical practice.[34] These communities are essentially 2-way streets of medical students learning through community immersion and the community learning through quality health care provision. Such community placements have demonstrated positive impacts on student competencies, including better clinical skills compared with those students learning in more traditional urban hospital-based settings.[35]

Student-run free clinics are another example of community-based medical education whereby health professional students offer free health services under the supervision of licensed health care professionals. The University of California, San Diego established the Student-Run Free Clinic Project to incorporate a curriculum of didactics in the philosophy and approach to working at a free clinic with taking on administrative and clinical roles in managing the clinic in the first 2 years of medical school followed by a primary care clerkship experience in their third and fourth years.[23] Loma Linda University has a program entitled "Street Medicine," in which students, under the supervision of licensed health care professionals, provide medical checkups, drug counseling, flu shots, and routine medical care to homeless populations of San Bernardino, California.[36]

Graduate medical education offered in MUAs range from electives to clerkships and longitudinal tracks or pathways. Some schools offer a 4-year longitudinal track directed toward health care provision in underserved areas with a curriculum that is immersed within the community, including community-based projects and didactic seminars.[37,38] The Albert Schweitzer Fellowship Program is an example of an extracurricular fellowship program funding leadership skills education and a health service project in the community.[39] Another example is the Brigham and Women's Hospital's residency in global health equity, established in 2004 as a combined 4-year internal medicine residency with an advanced study of public health.[40]

The international consortium of Training for Health Equity Network has established global institutions set forth to carry out an integration of health professional education to meet local needs and undertake research that is meaningful to the community.[41] This consortium evaluates the institutions through "The Framework for Social Accountability in Health Workforce Education," which helps health professional schools to restructure and evaluate their programs to comply with goals of attaining health equity worldwide.[41] In the Philippines, the socially accountable health professions education program, Ateneo de Zamboanga University School of Medicine, has implemented these approaches, yielding not only a 55% increase in the number of municipalities in Zamboanga with a doctor, but also a decline in the under-5 mortality from 89 per 1000 live births to 8 per 1000 since the initiation of the program.[42]

The Accreditation Council for Graduate Medical Education (ACGME) mandates all programs to teach trainees about health disparities. Interestingly, however, in a study exploring the perception of rheumatology fellows on their experience with health disparities education, it was noted that there was no formal health disparities curriculum and inadequate teaching of how to address health disparities in their patients.[37] When 5 focus groups were established in New York and Pennsylvania to query fellows' experiences with health disparities in their practices, 25 fellows in total endorsed feeling overwhelmingly frustrated with an inability to do enough for their patients, specifically not knowing what to do to address the disparities at hand.[43] In addition, fellows denied clear curriculum or training in addressing health disparities and reported lacking role models that regularly address health disparities.[43] These findings emphasize the importance of establishing a rheumatology-specific curriculum incorporated with service learning and community-based learning as approaches to formally train learners that will ultimate advocate for patients affected most by health disparities.

The Lupus Initiative's (TLI) Teaching Fellows in Lupus Project is a program through which rheumatology fellows provide seminars to frontline primary care providers on the diagnosis and management of lupus.[44] Since its inception in 2015, more than 900 nonrheumatologist providers have attended such seminars led by rheumatology fellows from 11 rheumatology programs in the United States and Canada. In reviewing responses from 660 providers asked to evaluate these seminars, reported gains were noted in knowledge, confidence in lupus competencies, and overall success of rheumatology fellows as lupus educators, specifically that 96% of responding providers were satisfied with the seminar content.[45] A similar program by TLI is the Expert Outreach Project, which provides online lupus education modules for rheumatology professionals to maintain rheumatology board certification (CARE:Lupus).[46]

RESEARCH IN MEDICALLY UNDERSERVED AREAS

Federal funding through programs like the Office of Minority Health Lupus Grants aim to begin the process of eliminating racial/ethnic disparities in adverse outcomes in rheumatic diseases, and specifically in lupus.[47] In one such project, researchers across the United States will be developing culturally and linguistically appropriate education programs to encourage recruitment and enrollment in clinical trials, as well as establishing education modules that are innovative and effective in improving confidence and provision of high-quality health care by health care providers.[47] Similarly, the National Institute of Arthritis and Musculoskeletal and Skin Diseases, with joint efforts from other National Institutes of Health components like the Office of Research on Minority Health, Office of Research on Women's Health, Office of Disease Prevention, and with the Centers for Disease Control and Prevention, the Arthritis Foundation, and the American College of Rheumatology express a commitment to addressing disparities of rheumatic disease in MUAs and HPSAs. Such programs encourage education and community-based research in MUAs and HPSAs to reduce barriers and improve health outcomes.

DISCUSSION

In rheumatology, education and work in underserved areas is particularly important because of the racial/ethnic and socioeconomic disparities that exist in different rheumatic diseases in disease onset, burden, disease course, response to therapies, and long-term outcomes. Despite this and the ACGME mandate on health disparities education, implementing such curricula into a training system remains a challenge. Where is the change needed? Who will monitor the outcomes and how will they do so? We acknowledge disparities warranting public health intervention that should be incorporated into medical education curriculum, but what social changes can be undertaken? The onus is on medical education institutions to train students to serve vulnerable communities to improve both health care access and the quality of medical school education.

Medical literature worldwide has repeatedly demonstrated a shortage of primary care and subspecialty providers in underserved regions. However, the value of education provided in and around MUAs and HPSAs is underrecognized. When health disparities are formally included in medical education curricula and the culture of medical education shifts to a service learning and community-based learning approach, patients and providers will reap the benefits. Improved health care capacity yields potential to improved health care quality services otherwise unattainable or difficult to attain, minority involvement in research will likely increase, and learners will possess a sense of understanding of health disparities that will allow for sustainable advocacy in the field with the ultimate goal of eliminating disparities altogether.

DISCLOSURES

Dr V.K. Sandhu and Dr D.M. Jose have no relevant financial disclosures. Dr C.H. Feldman receives funding from National Institutes of Health/National Institute of Arthritis and Musculoskeletal and Skin Diseases K23 AR071500, the Rheumatology Research Foundation Investigator Award, the Office of the Assistant Secretary for Health/Office of Minority Health 1 CPIMP181168-01-00, and the Brigham and Women's Hospital Health Equity Innovation Program. She has received research support from Bristol-Myers Squibb and from Pfizer Pharmaceuticals.

ACKNOWLEDGMENTS

This work was supported by NIH P30 AR072577 (VERITY).

REFERENCES

1. Institute of Medicine (US) Committee on Quality of Health Care in America. Crossing the quality Chasm: a new health system for the 21st century. Washington, DC: National Academies Press (US); 2001.
2. Global reference list of 100 core health indicators: working version 5. Geneva (Switzerland): World Health Organization; 2014. Available at: https://www.who.int/healthinfo/indicators/2018/en/. Accessed February 13, 2019.
3. Robeznieks A. Health equity commitment being embedded in DNA of AMA's work. AMA Association: Patient Support & Advocacy. 2019. Available at: https://www.ama-assn.org/delivering-care/patient-support-advocacy/health-equity-commitment-being-embedded-dna-ama-s-work?&utm_source=BulletinHealthCare&utm_medium=email&utm_term=012819&utm_content=NON-MEMBER&utm_campaign=article_alert-morning_rounds_daily&utm_uid=&utm_effort. Accessed February 13, 2019.
4. Ratcliff M, Burd C, Holder K, et al. Defining rural at the US Census Bureau. Washington, DC: ACSGEO- 1, US Census Bureau; 2016. Available at: https://www.census.gov/library/publications/2016/acs/acsgeo-1.html. Accessed February 10, 2019.
5. U.S. Census Bureau. Change in rural and urban population size: 1910-2010. Available at: https://www.census.gov/content/dam/Census/library/visualizations/2016/comm/acs-rural-urban.pdf. Accessed January 28, 2019.
6. FitzGerald JD, Benford L, Battistone M, et al. Regional distribution of adult rheumatologists. Arthritis Rheum 2013;65(12):3017–25.
7. ACGME. Rheumatology programs academic year 2015–2016. United States. Available at: https://apps.acgme.org/ads/Public/Reports/ReportRun?ReportId=8&CurrentYear=2017&SpecialtyId=&AcademicYearId=2015. Accessed February 1, 2019.
8. Battafarano DF, Ditmyer M, Bolster MB, et al. 2015 Workforce Study: supply and demand of adult rheumatology workforce, 2015-2030. Arthritis Care Res 2018;70(4):617–26.
9. Sacks JJ, Helmick CG, Luo YH, et al. Prevalence of and annual ambulatory health care visits for pediatric arthritis and other rheumatologic conditions in the United States in 2001–2004. Arthritis Rheum 2007;57:1439–45.
10. Address shortage of pediatric rheumatologists. Available at: https://www.arthritis.org/advocate/our-policy-priorities/access-to-care/increase-access-to-pediatric-rheumatologists. Accessed January 29, 2019.
11. American Association of Medical Colleges. 2018 update: the complexities of physician supply and demand: projections from 2016 to 2030. 2018. Available at: https://aamc-black.global.ssl.fastly.net/production/media/filer_public/85/d7/85d7b689-f417-4ef0-97fb-ecc129836829/aamc_2018_workforce_projections_update_april_11_2018.pdf. Accessed January 21, 2019.
12. MUA Find. Available at: https://data.hrsa.gov/tools/shortage-area/mua-find. Accessed January 2, 2019.
13. REACH 2018. Division of Nutrition, Physical Activity, and Obesity. 2018. Available at: https://www.cdc.gov/nccdphp/dnpao/state-local-programs/reach/current_programs/index.html. Accessed January 29, 2019.
14. Ferguson WJ, Cashman SB, Savageau JA, et al. Family medicine residency characteristics associated with practice in a health professions shortage area. Fam Med 2009;41(6):405–10.

15. Ko M, Edeksteub RA, Heslin KC, et al. Impact of the University of California Los Angeles/Charles R. Drew University medical education program on medical students' intention to practice in medically underserved areas. Acad Med 2005; 80(9):803–8.

16. Feldman CH, Hicks LS, Norton TL, et al. Assessing the need for improved access to rheumatology care: a survey of Massachusetts community health center medical directors. J Clin Rheumatol 2013;19(7):361–6.

17. Talley RC. Graduate medical education and rural health care. Acad Med 1990;65: 522–5.

18. Chase JL, LIsse JR, Brecht RM. Rheumatology in the 21st century - telemedicine leading the way. Arthritis Rheum 1995;38:R39.

19. Sanders PA. Cyberclinic in rheumatology. J R Coll Physicians Lond 1999;33: 400–1.

20. Lewtas J. Telemedicine in rheumatology. J Rheumatol 2001;28:1745–6.

21. Rothschild B. Telerheumatology: not ready for prime time. Intern Med J 2013;43: 468–9.

22. McDougall JA, Ferucci ED, Glover J, et al. Telerheumatology: a systematic review. Arthritis Care Res (Hoboken) 2017;69(10):1546–57.

23. Marcin JP, Ellis J, Mawis R, et al. Using telemedicine to provide pediatric subspecialty care to children with special health care needs in an underserved rural community. Pediatrics 2004;113(1):1–6.

24. Bullock DR, Vehe RK, Zhang L, et al. Telemedicine and other care models in pediatric rheumatology: an exploratory study of parents' perceptions of barriers to care and care preferences. Pediatr Rheumatol Online J 2017;15(1):55.

25. Arora S, Geppert CM, Kalishman S, et al. Academic health center management of chronic diseases through knowledge networks: Project ECHO. Acad Med 2007;82(2):154–60.

26. Vimalananda VG, Gupte G, Seraj SM, et al. Electronic consultations (e-consults) to improve access to specialty care: a systematic review and narrative synthesis. J Telemed Telecare 2015;21(6):323–30.

27. Eligibility for a waiver of the Exchange visitor two-year home-country physical presence requirement. Available at: https://travel.state.gov/content/travel/en/us-visas/study/exchange/waiver-of-the-exchange-visitor/eligibility.html. Accessed February 18, 2019.

28. National Resident Matching Program. Charting outcomes in the match, specialties matching service, appointment year 2018. Washington, DC: National Resident Matching Program; 2018.

29. Physician workforce: the special case of health centers and the National Health Service Corps. Am Fam Physician 2005;72(2):235.

30. Seifer SD. Service-learning: community-campus partnerships for health professions education. Acad Med 1998;73(3):273–7.

31. Gelmon SB, Holland BA, Shinnamon AF. Health Professions Schools in Service to the Nation. Conference Proceedings 1998. p. 8.

32. Palsdottir B, Neusy A, Reed G. Building the evidence base: networking innovative socially accountable medical education programs. Educ Health (Abingdon) 2008;8:177.

33. Larkins SL, Preston R, Matte MC, et al. Measuring social accountability in health professional education: development and international pilot testing of an evaluation framework. Med Teach 2013;35:32–5.

34. Magzoub ME, Schmidt HG. A taxonomy of community-based medical education. Acad Med 2000;75:699–707.

35. Chang LW, Kaye D, Muhwezi WW, et al. Perceptions and evaluation of a community-based education and service (COBES) program in Uganda. Med Teach 2011;33:e9–15.
36. Street Medicine, Loma Linda University Health. Available at: https://caps.llu.edu/volunteer-now/street-medicine. Accessed February 18, 2019.
37. Huang W, Malinow A. Curriculum and evaluation results of a third-year medical student longitudinal pathway on underserved care. Teach Learn Med 2010; 22(2):123–30.
38. Smucny J, Beatty P, Grant W, et al. An evaluation of the Rural Medical Education Program of the State University of New York Upstate Medical University, 1990-2003. Acad Med 2005;80(8):733–8.
39. Albert Schweitzer Fellowship. Improving Health. Developing leaders. Creating change. Available at: http://www.schweitzerfellowship.org/about/. Accessed January 15, 2019.
40. Doris and Howard Hiatt residency in global health equity and internal medicine. Available at: https://www.brighamandwomens.org/medicine/global-health-equity/hiatt-residency-in-global-health-equity-and-internal-medicine. Accessed February 18, 2019.
41. Training for health equity around the world. Available at: https://thenetcommunity.org. Accessed December 18, 2018.
42. Cristobal F, Worley P. Can medical education in poor rural areas be cost-effective and sustainable: the case of the Ateneo de Zamboanga University School of Medicine. Rural Remote Health 2012;12:1835.
43. Blanco I, Gonzalez C. Current rheumatology fellows experiences with health disparities and disparity education: a qualitative study [abstract]. Arthritis Rheumatol 2018;70(suppl 10). Available at: https://acrabstracts.org/abstract/current-rheumatology-fellows-experiences-with-health-disparities-and-disparity-education-a-qualitative-study. Accessed January 30, 2019.
44. Caron A, Lim SS, Rene L, et al. Teaching fellows in lupus: rheumatology fellows are successful educators in improving lupus recognition by frontline healthcare providers. Arthritis Rheumatol 2015;2015:67.
45. Fellows project: demystifying lupus. Available at: https://thelupusinitiative.org/educators-students/seminars/. Accessed February 18, 2019.
46. St. Clair EW. The ACR's lupus initiative expands training, Educational Resources. 2015. Available at: https://www.the-rheumatologist.org/article/the-acrs-lupus-initiative-expands-training-educational-resources/. Accessed February 18, 2019.
47. US Department of Health and Human Services Office of Minority Health, Lupus Grants. Available at: https://minorityhealth.hhs.gov/omh/browse.aspx?lvl=2&lvlid=62. Accessed January 30, 2019.

Addressing Health Disparities in Medical Education and Clinical Practice

Irene Blanco, MD, MS[a,*], Nevena Barjaktarovic, MD[a],
Cristina M. Gonzalez, MD, MEd[b]

KEYWORDS

- Health disparities • Cultural competency • Underserved populations
- Graduate medical education • Rheumatology fellowship

KEY POINTS

- Health disparities are pervasive in all medical specialties including rheumatology.
- Medical education interventions can help to increase a provider's knowledge in terms of the issues and provide more culturally competent care.
- Although several interventions are discussed, little is currently being done in rheumatology. Therefore, the authors suggest ways that training programs can address these topics in their curricula.

INTRODUCTION

In 2003, the National Academy of Medicine (NAM), then known as the Institute of Medicine, issued a report that reverberated throughout all of medicine. The report, titled *Unequal Treatment: Confronting Racial and Ethnic Disparities in Health Care*, culled together years of research elucidating that patients who were poor and/or from racial and ethnic minorities were receiving unequal care and had worse outcomes as compared with other American populations. They emphasized that health disparities were pervasive and not relegated to one particular field. Although differences could in part be caused by socioeconomic status (SES), it was evident that for racial and ethnic minorities, these disparities remained after controlling for income and other SES related factors.[1]

The cause of disparities is multifactorial. Although the NAM report uncovered some patient-associated factors contributing to disparities, such as patient treatment

[a] Department of Medicine - Rheumatology, Albert Einstein College of Medicine, 1300 Morris Park Avenue, Forchh 107N, Bronx, NY 10461, USA; [b] Department of Medicine - Hospital Medicine, Albert Einstein College of Medicine, Montefiore Medical Center, 1825 Eastchester Road, DOM 2-76, Bronx, NY 10461, USA
* Corresponding author.
E-mail address: irene.blanco@einstein.yu.edu

Rheum Dis Clin N Am 46 (2020) 179–191
https://doi.org/10.1016/j.rdc.2019.09.012
0889-857X/20/© 2019 Elsevier Inc. All rights reserved.

preferences and mistrust in the medical system, the effects of these were low. They highlighted that most health disparities arise from the health care system itself in addition to individual factors stemming from the clinical encounter. To address these disparities, they outlined multiple interventions including the collection of outcomes data by race and ethnicity, the need to follow evidence-based medicine, and to perform continuous quality improvement to ensure that patients are receiving equitable care. Regarding education, they recommended providers increase their knowledge as to the cause of health disparities in addition to the integration of cross-cultural training into various medical curricula.[1,2] In response, medical schools and residencies are incorporating disparities education into curricula with the goal that training future providers will result in improved patient outcomes. In this review we highlight the efforts in graduate medical education and delineate the nascent efforts in rheumatology where we hope to inspire fellow medical educators to address disparities within their individual programs.

HEALTH DISPARITIES IN RHEUMATOLOGY

Currently, the Centers for Disease Control and Prevention define health disparities as the "preventable differences in the burden of disease, injury, violence or in opportunities to achieve optimal health by socially disadvantaged groups."[3] Some persist in defining health disparities as health outcomes differences among populations because of biologic factors, such as genetics. However, as pointed out by Dehlendorf and colleagues,[4] from "a social justice perspective, we believe it is most important to focus on those differences which society has a role in creating, and therefore has the greatest potential to ameliorate." Therefore it is critical to look within our fields to understand the nature and causes of health disparities.

When analyzing rheumatology, we likewise find that several conditions are fraught with disparities, having been best described is systemic lupus erythematosus (SLE). In the United States, SLE disproportionately affects patients of color; it has a higher incidence and prevalence in black, Hispanic, Asian, and Native American/American Indian populations.[5,6] Although disparities in lupus have been described sporadically in the past, the Lupus in Minority Populations, Nature versus Nurture (LUMINA) study has been instrumental in deeply investigating the nature of these health disparities particularly in black and Hispanic patients.[7–9] LUMINA has found that despite there being some genetic differences associated with various HLA-DRB alleles, overall black and Hispanic patients tend to present with higher disease activity at baseline.[7,10] LUMINA has also found that they tend to present with SLE at younger ages and have more extensive disease activity, organ damage, and higher mortality rates.[11,12] In addition poverty was found to be associated with higher disease activity, particularly for black patients.[13] Although the LUMINA cohort has been instrumental at describing disparities in patients with SLE, their findings have been replicated in multiple other studies and cohorts.[14–17]

Despite the extensive data available regarding disparities in SLE, it is certainly not the only condition where they have been reported. Given the cost and accessibility of the biologic disease-modifying antirheumatic drugs (DMARDs), and the extent of disability from rheumatoid arthritis (RA), it is another condition where scholars have sought to understand the nature of the observed disparities. In several cohorts, patients from racial and ethnic minorities, patients with lower SES scores, and patients with limited English proficiency (LEP) tend to have poorer pain scores, increased disability, and worse overall outcomes.[18–21] The nature of the disparities in RA is multifactorial and they arise from patient, provider, and systems-based issues. On the patient side, ethnic minority patients and those with lower levels of education often opted for less aggressive RA therapy.[22,23] Adherence, particularly as it relates to systems issues, also likely contributes to disparities, where those with financial difficulties, those uninsured, and those with low health literacy and LEP have difficulty taking their prescribed treatment regimens for various reasons.[24] On the provider side, there are delays to the initiation of DMARDs in nonwhite patients and those of lower SES levels.[25,26] Regarding systems issues, a survey of primary care providers shows that lack of rheumatologists available to see Medicaid and Medicare patients significantly impacts care given these providers are uncomfortable initiating DMARDs without the support of their rheumatology colleagues.[27]

Osteoarthritis (OA) is not only the most common form of arthritis in the United States, it is also the primary cause of disability.[28,29] Given the impact of arthritis in the United States it is imperative that one understand and recognize the cause of disparities among patients with OA. Black patients have higher rates of OA compared with white patients.[30] However, despite having significantly higher rates of disease, black patients have much lower rates of arthroplasty.[31–33] Skinner and colleagues[31] found that income, in addition to geographic location, contributed to the racial disparities seen in analysis of Medicare beneficiaries. As in the case for RA, the causes are likely multifactorial. Patients from ethnic minorities may fear poor outcomes from arthroplasty and therefore elect not to undergo the procedure.[34] This fear may be borne out by the fact that racial and ethnic minorities tend to undergo arthroplasty at low-volume institutions, which often have poorer outcomes with increased postoperative infections and increased revision rates. These poorer outcomes may confirm community members expectations of poor outcomes, leading them to avoid such procedures, thereby perpetuating the cycle of disparity.[35–37]

Although OA, RA, and SLE have much data concerning existing health disparities, more data are beginning to emerge from other conditions, such as gout and psoriatic arthritis.[37,38] Elucidating health disparities is incredibly important but mere descriptions do not suffice. The key to equitable care is the implementation of interventions that seek to reduce and ultimately eliminate disparities. One way to ameliorate disparities, as suggested by the NAM, has been to educate providers during their training with the expectation that educated providers are empowered to address health disparities within their own patient populations.

MANDATES FOR ADDRESSING HEALTH DISPARITIES IN GRADUATE MEDICAL EDUCATION

Many medical schools are addressing disparities and culturally sensitive care to varying degrees within their curricula, yet there is no assurance that any given fellow would have participated in such a curriculum. In addition, more than 45% of the incoming rheumatology fellows in 2019 are foreign medical graduates. Therefore, even if their medical schools addressed disparities, it may not have been in terms of the US context.[39] To reach all future rheumatologists this content must be addressed within the realm of graduate medical education.

Because of the pervasive and persistent nature of health disparities, the Accreditation Council for Graduate Medical Education (ACGME) through their Clinical Learning Environment Review initiative has mandated that any ACGME accredited program must perform the following[40]:

1. Residents/fellows and faculty members receive education on identifying and reducing health care disparities relevant to the patient population served by the clinical site (HQ5).

2. Residents/fellows and faculty members receive training in cultural competency relevant to the patient population served by the clinical site (HQ5).
3. Residents/fellows and faculty members know the clinical site's priorities for addressing health care disparities (HQ5).
4. Residents/fellows are engaged in quality improvement activities addressing health care disparities for the vulnerable populations served by the clinical site.

In addition, as of July 1, 2019, the common program requirements for ACGME accredited programs mandate that[41]:

The mission of institutions participating in graduate medical education is to improve the health of the public. Each community has health needs that vary based upon location and demographics. Programs must understand the social determinants of health of the populations they serve and incorporate them in the design and implementation of the program curriculum, with the ultimate goal of addressing these needs and health disparities.

Despite clear mandates from the ACGME, it is unclear to what extent residencies and fellowships have implemented their own curricula. A survey of 954 US residents across 29 states showed that health disparities knowledge did not improve with each postgraduate year.[42] In addition, in the last round of Clinical Learning Environment Review site visits, although house officers were able to identify which of their populations were most at risk for health disparities, few programs seemed to have a formal structure to address disparities. It was uncommon that house officers, faculty members, and program directors were involved in these efforts in any substantive way.[43] Additional challenges to house staff training have been: (1) informal cultural competency training that often does not address the populations served by the programs surveyed, (2) lack of standardized curricula, and (3) poorly perceived self-efficacy to discuss disease-specific (eg, diabetes) disparities with patients and to care for LEP patients and families.[43-46] According to a survey of internal medicine residency program directors, the most common barriers to the implementation of a health disparities curriculum were: (1) lack of faculty expertise, (2) not enough faculty that understand how to assess resident's cultural competency skills, (3) not enough institutional resources, and (4) not enough time.[47]

To address these challenges, investigators have sought the perspective of intended learners. Perspectives of preferred methods to learn about health disparities include didactics, experiential learning, and skill development in addressing disparities directly relevant to their clinical practice.[45] In addition, investigators suggest promoting a patient-centered approach, highlighting best practices (eg, in interpreter use), and using a combined approach of dedicated time for health disparities instruction and integrating instruction into existing small group discussions and active learning opportunities.[42,44,46] Frameworks and curricula published in the literature incorporate these opportunities for instruction while addressing perceived challenges. We describe aspects of this work to highlight opportunities for innovation in rheumatology fellowship curricula.

RESOURCES FOR PROGRAMS TO ADDRESS DISPARITIES
Framework

The Society of General Internal Medicine's Health Equity Commission (SGIM HEC-formerly known as the SGIM Disparities Task Force) suggests that the goal of health disparities curricula should be that learners not only develop a personal commitment to ending health disparities, but that they also understand their own roles contributing to an inequitable system. Therefore, to create instruction addressing the multiple contributors to health and health care disparities, they recommend that any such curricula have these three key learning objectives[44]:

1. Understand attitudes, such as mistrust, subconscious (implicit) bias, and stereotyping that practitioners and/or patients may bring to the clinical encounter.
2. Attain knowledge of the existence and magnitude of health disparities, including the multifactorial etiologies of and the multiple solutions required to eliminate them.
3. Acquire the skills to effectively communicate and negotiate across cultures, including trust-building and the use of key tools to improve cross-cultural communication.

These learning objectives, although targeted and measurable, are still broad and lend themselves to various lecture-based and active, experiential learning methods. This allows them to be customized for various settings including the incorporation into a graduate medical education curriculum, and necessary faculty development.

Curricula: Faculty Development

The importance of faculty role modeling cannot be underestimated; however, there is a reported dearth of faculty expertise in addressing these issues.[47] Therefore the SGIM-HEC published a "train the trainer" guide.[48] Full details are available as an online resource that can guide faculty development efforts to equip faculty with the knowledge and skills to effectively facilitate health disparities instruction.[49] The five modules, along with a brief description of each, are listed in **Table 1**. Modules cover systemic and individual contributions to health disparities, such as social determinants of health and provider implicit bias.[48,49] Finally, an innovative approach that may not only capitalize on existing faculty expertise, but also addresses multiple ACGME competencies (systems-based practice and practice-based learning) is to apply a health equity lens to quality improvement efforts.[50] Aysola and Myers[50] describe a four-step framework that guides medical educators' efforts to embed equity into existing quality improvement instruction and projects (**Table 2**).

Curricula: Graduate Medical Education

Curricula providing didactic and experiential learning that strive to incorporate local health disparities and engagement with the local community can maximize the relevance of the content for the intended learners, a central tenet to adult learning theory.[51] Patow and colleagues[52] reviewed experiential learning opportunities that can be adapted to an individual fellowship's local environment. Opportunities included community tours, films, collaboration, and simulated encounters, among others. Poverty simulations have demonstrated increased understanding of the influence of poverty and the social determinants of health on health and wellness, and are delivered in 2 hours to an entire cohort of fellows.[53]

In addition to raising awareness of the contexts of some patients' lived experiences, programs such as these provide instruction in advocacy to empower learners to address health disparities.[53] As with faculty development, others in residency education have applied a health equity lens to quality improvement education and used the Plan-Do-Study-Act cycle in didactic and problem-based learning related to local health disparities.[54] Finally, Noriea and colleagues[55] developed an eight-session curriculum delivered over 2 years for internal medicine residents. Broadly, this curriculum uses didactics, small group discussions, learner presentations, and experiential learning within the local community and is extensively described in their publication. An outline of these interventions is found in **Table 3**.

Modules	Content Areas
Table 1 **Overview of the train the trainer guide: health disparities education program from the Society of General Internal Medicine Disparities Task Force**	
Module 1. Disparities foundations	Review of disparities data Role of social determinants Role of health care Role of provider-patient encounter Resources for updating disparities information
Module 2. Teaching disparities in the clinical setting	Challenges to teaching in the clinical setting (hidden curriculum, institutional dynamics) Suggestions for working with skeptical learners (eg, reasons for resistance, model and recognize good behavior, demonstrate knowledge and skills) Five cases (limited English proficiency, medical mistakes, limited literacy, stereotyping, informed consent)
Module 3. Disparities beyond the clinical setting	Sample exercises: increasing awareness of self and others Small group teaching triggers Large group lectures: trust, disparities Addressing bias Sample cases, vignettes, and video resources
Module 4. Teaching about disparities through community involvement	Description and overview of the US health care system Introduction to community Worlds apart: discussion of mistrust of health care and racism and how they contribute to health care disparities, particularly in some African American communities Community as a positive force
Module 5. Curriculum evaluation	Program evaluation, design features of an evaluation study that allow investigator to: draw conclusions about specific instance, and identify threats to reliability and validity

Data from Society of General Internal Medicine (SGIM). A Train the Trainer Guide: Health Disparities Education, 2008. Available at: https://www.sgim.org/File%20Library/SGIM/Communities/Education/Resources/SGIM-DTFES-Health-Disparities-Training-Guide.pdf. Accessed Feb 21 2019.

CURRENT EFFORTS WITHIN RHEUMATOLOGY

In 2017, the American College of Rheumatology approved the creation of a dedicated disparities educational program so that this topic could be formally incorporated into the core rheumatology curriculum. These efforts are currently being led by our group. Despite extensive data regarding the prevalence of health disparities within rheumatology, little is known in terms of whether our fellowships are actually addressing disparities. To investigate this, we conducted a small study during the 2013 New York City Rheumatology Objective Structured Clinical Exam; our findings suggested there is some fellowship disparities education. Fellows were evaluated on how well they were able to assess a standardized patient's (SP) social determinants of health at one station where they had to determine that a patient with RA had stopped their biologic medications secondary to finances. Fellows training in programs located in lower income neighborhoods were determined by the SPs to have better assessed the SP's finances ($P = .003$) and trended toward being less judgmental toward the SP's lack of resources ($P = .071$).[56] It is unknown if this is secondary to exposure to an underresourced population or if the fellows that performed well actually had disparities education.

Table 2
Overview of quality improvement framework to address health disparities proposed by Aysola and Myers

Step	Content Area
Step 1. Define terms and concepts	Review of the basic terms and concepts related to health equity Explaining distinction between HCDs and HDs Reducing HCD: should be initial focus within QI efforts
Step 2. Understand and disseminate the current knowledge of HCDs in field	Set of strategies that medical educators can use to engage residents/fellows to address HCDs, using a two-step method: (1) raising faculty awareness of HD/HCD relevant in their clinical field; (2) develop a plan of dissemination of this information to colleagues and trainees
Step 3. Identify HCDs locally and apply QI methods to address them	Reviewing potential sources and methods for obtaining/analyzing data to determine whether and if so, why an equity gap may exist in an institution Review strategies for and share examples of applying classic QI methods to address identified disparities
Step 4. Evaluate every QI effort for the potential equity angle	Independent from previous steps Addressing how every QI effort provides an opportunity to consider health equity

Abbreviations: HCD, health care disparity; HD, health disparity; QI, quality improvement.
Data from Aysola J, Myers JS. Integrating Training in Quality Improvement and Health Equity in Graduate Medical Education: Two Curricula for the Price of One. Acad Med 2018;93(1):31-34.

To better understand this issue, and to serve as our needs assessment for curricular development, we held a series of focus groups with rheumatology fellows over the course of 2018. Preliminary data show findings similar to those seen in other graduate medical education programs: fellows are given little formal education on health disparities and are often overwhelmed by their patients' needs and typically have little (and occasionally poor) role-modeling in addressing disparities and culturally responsive care. Despite these challenges, many participating fellows expressed eagerness to learn how to better address these issues and help their patients.[57]

Although we are at the early stages of curricular development, based on the frameworks noted previously, we have begun creating sessions that we think programs directors will be able to modify and incorporate into their curricula. As part of our modules we developed a community tour for our rheumatology fellows. Although the Bronx is incredibly vibrant and has several noted tourist destinations, it also has some of the worst health outcomes in all of New York. Therefore we devised a tour to provide the fellows with some context regarding those health outcomes and to help them better understand the neighborhoods of the Bronx and the people living within them.[58,59] In addition, we have begun to incorporate reflective writing sessions into our protected didactic time so that the fellows can articulate the challenges they are facing taking care of our populations. These reflections serve two purposes: they provide opportunities to identify and implement solutions, and so that as a program director (IB), I too am aware of the challenges that they and our patients are facing, and tailor instruction as necessary.

SUMMARY

Several organizations have recommended formal training in health disparities and the social determinants of health.[1,60] Although several medical schools and residency

Table 3
Overview of several educational methods and interventions in health disparity education

Reference	Educational Method/Model	Brief Description	Topics Covered
Patow et al,[52] 2016	Experiential education	Educational models developed for residents, fellows, and faculty with goal to improve understanding of cultural diversity and health care disparity Various models used, including simulation scenarios, community tours, house calls, cultural films, and so forth	Ethnic and cultural diversity Cultural competence in health care Community advocacy Social determinants of health Ethnic foods, cultural goods, and traditional remedies
Paul et al,[53] 2009	Medical-legal partnerships	Education of medical students and residents, by lawyers, how to address patients' legal needs Promotes physician role in advocating for housing and government benefits for their patients	Family advocacy Legal assistance for medical patients Medical-legal partnership
Benson et al,[54] 2018	Quality improvement health disparity initiative	Educational initiative designed to increase resident awareness of prevalent health disparities in the community delivered through PDSA framework, divided into 2 cycles Cycles were organized through either didactic sessions (PDSA cycle I) or small group discussion format (PDSA cycle II)	General health disparity Diabetes-related health disparity, diabetes self-management and education
Ross et al,[48] 2010	"Train the Trainer" curricula	A 5-module curricula on health disparity in various settings and social determinants of health, designated to educate faculty through didactics, small group sessions, case-based lectures, and so forth	Disparity foundations Teaching disparities in the clinical setting Disparities beyond the clinical setting Teaching about disparity through community involvement Curriculum evaluation
Noriea et al,[55] 2017	Lecture-based curricula	General health disparity 2-y curricula for internal medicine residents, delivered through didactics sessions and experiential learning (assigned videos) and case discussions	Social determinants of health Environmental determinants of health Patient-provider interaction Patient advocacy Disparities in research Language, acculturation, and immigrant health

Abbreviation: PDSA, plan-do-study-act.

programs have incorporated this training, the design and implementation of said curricula have been quite varied.[61] Given that these curricula are so varied in their design and implementation, it is difficult to study their long-term outcomes making it unclear if medical education interventions are sufficient in addressing population-level health disparities.[61–63] Therefore, medical education interventions that are rigorously evaluated, in addition to interventions that address systematic causes of disparities, are needed to affect the overarching disparities seen in our patient populations.[61,64,65]

Health and health care disparities are pervasive throughout medicine and rheumatology is no exception. Those that are most affected by the rheumatic diseases tend to be from typically marginalized and underserved populations. For us to best care for our patients, we must extend our focus beyond the pathogenesis and potential treatments for each rheumatic condition. We must educate ourselves so that we can partner with our patients, advocate on their behalf, and address disparities as part of our routine clinical and teaching duties. All specialties must come together to address the disparities in their respective fields so that we can contribute to ultimately achieving health equity. Educating fellows is a vital step in achieving this goal.

DISCLOSURE

None of the authors listed have any relevant financial disclosures.

REFERENCES

1. Smedley BD, Stith AY, Nelson AR, Institute of Medicine (U.S.), Committee on Understanding and Eliminating Racial and Ethnic Disparities in Health Care. Unequal treatment: confronting racial and ethnic disparities in health care. Washington, DC: National Academy Press; 2003.
2. Betancourt JR, Maina AW. The Institute of Medicine report "unequal treatment": implications for academic health centers. Mt Sinai J Med 2004;71(5):314–21.
3. Centers for Disease Control and Prevention. Health disparities. Available at: https://www.cdc.gov/aging/disparities/index.htm. Accessed April 3, 2019.
4. Dehlendorf C, Bryant AS, Huddleston HG, et al. Health disparities: definitions and measurements. Am J Obstet Gynecol 2010;202(3):212–3.
5. Izmirly PM, Wan I, Sahl S, et al. The incidence and prevalence of systemic lupus erythematosus in New York County (Manhattan), New York: the Manhattan lupus surveillance program. Arthritis Rheumatol 2017;69(10):2006–17.
6. Peschken CA, Esdaile JM. Rheumatic diseases in North America's indigenous peoples. Semin Arthritis Rheum 1999;28(6):368–91.
7. Reveille JD, Moulds JM, Ahn C, et al. Systemic lupus erythematosus in three ethnic groups: I. The effects of HLA class II, C4, and CR1 alleles, socioeconomic factors, and ethnicity at disease onset. LUMINA Study Group. Lupus in minority populations, nature versus nurture. Arthritis Rheum 1998;41(7):1161–72.
8. Petri M. The effect of race on incidence and clinical course in systemic lupus erythematosus: the Hopkins Lupus Cohort. J Am Med Womens Assoc (1972) 1998; 53(1):9–12.
9. Petri M, Perez-Gutthann S, Longenecker JC, et al. Morbidity of systemic lupus erythematosus: role of race and socioeconomic status. Am J Med 1991;91(4): 345–53.
10. Alarcon GS, Roseman J, Bartolucci AA, et al. Systemic lupus erythematosus in three ethnic groups: II. Features predictive of disease activity early in its course.

LUMINA Study Group. Lupus in minority populations, nature versus nurture. Arthritis Rheum 1998;41(7):1173–80.

11. Alarcon GS, Friedman AW, Straaton KV, et al. Systemic lupus erythematosus in three ethnic groups: III. A comparison of characteristics early in the natural history of the LUMINA cohort. LUpus in MInority populations: NAture vs. Nurture. Lupus 1999;8(3):197–209.

12. Alarcon GS, McGwin G Jr, Bastian HM, et al. Systemic lupus erythematosus in three ethnic groups. VII [correction of VIII]. Predictors of early mortality in the LUMINA cohort. LUMINA Study Group. Arthritis Rheum 2001;45(2):191–202.

13. Alarcon GS, McGwin G Jr, Sanchez ML, et al. Systemic lupus erythematosus in three ethnic groups. XIV. Poverty, wealth, and their influence on disease activity. Arthritis Rheum 2004;51(1):73–7.

14. Demas KL, Costenbader KH. Disparities in lupus care and outcomes. Curr Opin Rheumatol 2009;21(2):102–9.

15. Anderson E, Nietert PJ, Kamen DL, et al. Ethnic disparities among patients with systemic lupus erythematosus in South Carolina. J Rheumatol 2008;35(5): 819–25.

16. Mok CC. Racial difference in the prognosis of lupus nephritis. Nephrology (Carlton) 2010;15(4):480–1.

17. Clowse ME, Grotegut C. Racial and ethnic disparities in the pregnancies of women with systemic lupus erythematosus. Arthritis Care Res (Hoboken) 2016; 68(10):1567–72.

18. Bruce B, Fries JF, Murtagh KN. Health status disparities in ethnic minority patients with rheumatoid arthritis: a cross-sectional study. J Rheumatol 2007;34(7): 1475–9.

19. Harrison MJ, Farragher TM, Clarke AM, et al. Association of functional outcome with both personal- and area-level socioeconomic inequalities in patients with inflammatory polyarthritis. Arthritis Rheum 2009;61(10):1297–304.

20. Barton JL, Trupin L, Schillinger D, et al. Racial and ethnic disparities in disease activity and function among persons with rheumatoid arthritis from university-affiliated clinics. Arthritis Care Res (Hoboken) 2011;63(9):1238–46.

21. Greenberg JD, Spruill TM, Shan Y, et al. Racial and ethnic disparities in disease activity in patients with rheumatoid arthritis. Am J Med 2013;126(12):1089–98.

22. Constantinescu F, Goucher S, Weinstein A, et al. Racial disparities in treatment preferences for rheumatoid arthritis. Med Care 2009;47(3):350–5.

23. Constantinescu F, Goucher S, Weinstein A, et al. Understanding why rheumatoid arthritis patient treatment preferences differ by race. Arthritis Rheum 2009;61(4): 413–8.

24. Garcia Popa-Lisseanu MG, Greisinger A, Richardson M, et al. Determinants of treatment adherence in ethnically diverse, economically disadvantaged patients with rheumatic disease. J Rheumatol 2005;32(5):913–9.

25. Suarez-Almazor ME, Berrios-Rivera JP, Cox V, et al. Initiation of disease-modifying antirheumatic drug therapy in minority and disadvantaged patients with rheumatoid arthritis. J Rheumatol 2007;34(12):2400–7.

26. Solomon DH, Yelin E, Katz JN, et al. Treatment of rheumatoid arthritis in the Medicare Current Beneficiary Survey. Arthritis Res Ther 2013;15(2):R43.

27. Feldman CH, Hicks LS, Norton TL, et al. Assessing the need for improved access to rheumatology care: a survey of Massachusetts community health center medical directors. J Clin Rheumatol 2013;19(7):361–6.

28. Centers for Disease Control and Prevention. Prevalence and most common causes of disability among adults—United States, 2005. MMWR Morb Mortal Wkly Rep 2009;58(16):421–6.

29. Vina ER, Kwoh CK. Epidemiology of osteoarthritis: literature update. Curr Opin Rheumatol 2018;30(2):160–7.

30. Dillon CF, Rasch EK, Gu Q, et al. Prevalence of knee osteoarthritis in the United States: arthritis data from the Third National Health and Nutrition Examination Survey 1991-94. J Rheumatol 2006;33(11):2271–9.

31. Skinner J, Weinstein JN, Sporer SM, et al. Racial, ethnic, and geographic disparities in rates of knee arthroplasty among Medicare patients. N Engl J Med 2003; 349(14):1350–9.

32. Pierce TP, Elmallah RK, Lavernia CJ, et al. Racial disparities in lower extremity arthroplasty outcomes and use. Orthopedics 2015;38(12):e1139–46.

33. Goodman SM, Parks ML, McHugh K, et al. Disparities in outcomes for African Americans and whites undergoing total knee arthroplasty: a systematic literature review. J Rheumatol 2016;43(4):765–70.

34. Bradley LA, Deutsch G, McKendree-Smith NL, et al. Pain-related beliefs and affective pain responses: implications for ethnic disparities in preferences for joint arthroplasty. J Rheumatol 2005;32(6):1149–52.

35. Adelani MA, Keller MR, Barrack RL, et al. The impact of hospital volume on racial differences in complications, readmissions, and emergency department visits following total joint arthroplasty. J Arthroplasty 2018;33(2):309–315 e320.

36. Chen JC, Shaw JD, Ma Y, et al. The role of the hospital and health care system characteristics in readmissions after major surgery in California. Surgery 2016; 159(2):381–8.

37. Figaro MK, Williams-Russo P, Allegrante JP. Expectation and outlook: the impact of patient preference on arthritis care among African Americans. J Ambul Care Manage 2005;28(1):41–8.

38. Kerr GS, Qaiyumi S, Richards J, et al. Psoriasis and psoriatic arthritis in African-American patients: the need to measure disease burden. Clin Rheumatol 2015; 34(10):1753–9.

39. National Resident Matching Program. Results and data: specialties matching service. Available at: www.nrmp.org. Accessed April 3, 2019.

40. Accreditation Council for Graduate Medical Education. Available at: http://www.acgme.org/What-We-Do/Initiatives/Clinical-Learning-Environment-Review-CLER. Accessed April 3, 2019.

41. Accreditation Council for Graduate Medical Education. Common Program Requirements 2019. Available at: https://www.acgme.org/What-We-Do/Accreditation/Common-Program-Requirements. Accessed April 3, 2019.

42. Marshall JK, Cooper LA, Green AR, et al. Residents' attitude, knowledge, and perceived preparedness toward caring for patients from diverse sociocultural backgrounds. Health Equity 2017;1(1):43–9.

43. Accreditation Council for Graduate Medical Education. CLER National Report of Findings 2018 Executive Report. Available at: https://www.acgme.org/Portals/0/PDFs/CLER/CLER_2018_Executive_Summary_DIGITAL_081418.pdf. Accessed April 3, 2019.

44. Smith WR, Betancourt JR, Wynia MK, et al. Recommendations for teaching about racial and ethnic disparities in health and health care. Ann Intern Med 2007; 147(9):654–65.

45. Taylor YJ, Davis ME, Mohanan S, et al. Awareness of racial disparities in diabetes among primary care residents and preparedness to discuss disparities with patients. J Racial Ethn Health Disparities 2019;6(2):237–44.

46. Hernandez RG, Cowden JD, Moon M, et al. Predictors of resident satisfaction in caring for limited English proficient families: a multisite study. Acad Pediatr 2014; 14(2):173–80.

47. Cardinal LJ, Maldonado M, Fried ED. A national survey to evaluate graduate medical education in disparities and limited English proficiency: a report from the AAIM Diversity and Inclusion Committee. Am J Med 2016;129(1):117–25.

48. Ross PT, Wiley Cene C, Bussey-Jones J, et al. A strategy for improving health disparities education in medicine. J Gen Intern Med 2010;25(Suppl 2):S160–3.

49. Society of General Internal Medicine. A train the trainer guide: health disparities education. 2008. Available at: https://www.sgim.org/File%20Library/SGIM/Communities/Education/Resources/SGIM-DTFES-Health-Disparities-Training-Guide.pdf. Accessed February 21, 2019.

50. Aysola J, Myers JS. Integrating training in quality improvement and health equity in graduate medical education: two curricula for the price of one. Acad Med 2018;93(1):31–4.

51. Merriam SCR, Baumgartner L. Learning in adulthood: a comprehensive guide. San Francisco (CA): John Wiley & Sons, Inc.; 2007.

52. Patow C, Bryan D, Johnson G, et al. Who's in our neighborhood? Healthcare disparities experiential education for residents. Ochsner J 2016;16(1):41–4.

53. Paul E, Fullerton DF, Cohen E, et al. Medical-legal partnerships: addressing competency needs through lawyers. J Grad Med Educ 2009;1(2):304–9.

54. Benson BL, Ha M, Stansfield RB, et al. Health disparities educational initiative for residents. Ochsner J 2018;18(2):151–8.

55. Noriea AH, Redmond N, Weil RA, et al. Development of a multifaceted health disparities curriculum for medical residents. Fam Med 2017;49(10):796–802.

56. Blanco I, Sutaria R, Aizer J, et al. Addressing medical non-adherence from lack of finances in an observed structured clinical exam of rheumatology fellows [abstract]. Arthritis Rheum 2015;67(suppl 10).

57. Blanco I, Gonzalez CM. Rheumatology fellows experiences with health disparities and disparity education: a qualitative study [abstract]. Arthritis Rheum 2018; 70(suppl 10).

58. Lichtenstein C, de la Torre D, Falusi O, et al. Using a community bus tour for pediatric residents to increase their knowledge of health disparities. Acad Pediatr 2018;18(6):717–9.

59. Blanco I, Archer-Dyer H. An innovative pilot educational program to inform rheumatology fellows about the population of the Bronx: issues affecting and resources available to the community [abstract]. Arthritis Rheum 2018; 70(suppl 10).

60. Marmot M. Closing the health gap in a generation: the work of the Commission on Social Determinants of Health and its recommendations. Glob Health Promot 2009;(Suppl 1):23–7.

61. Gard LA, Peterson J, Miller C, et al. Social determinants of health training in U.S. primary care residency programs: a scoping review. Acad Med 2019;94(1): 135–43.

62. Truong M, Paradies Y, Priest N. Interventions to improve cultural competency in healthcare: a systematic review of reviews. BMC Health Serv Res 2014;14:99.

63. Jongen CS, McCalman J, Bainbridge RG. The implementation and evaluation of health promotion services and programs to improve cultural competency: a systematic scoping review. Front Public Health 2017;5:24.
64. Betancourt JR, Green AR. Commentary: linking cultural competence training to improved health outcomes: perspectives from the field. Acad Med 2010;85(4): 583–5.
65. Clarke AR, Goddu AP, Nocon RS, et al. Thirty years of disparities intervention research: what are we doing to close racial and ethnic gaps in health care? Med Care 2013;51(11):1020–6.

Printed and bound by CPI Group (UK) Ltd, Croydon, CR0 4YY

08/05/2025

01864746-0009